PRAISE FOR *WIRED FOR*

M000095761

"Only a few people have the courage, vision, and love for humanity to be pioneers. Susan Smith Jones is one of them. Fortunately, where pioneers like her are willing to go, many people can follow more confidently. If your goals are health, happiness, and a meaningful life, *Wired for High-Level Wellness* is for you."

—BRIAN BOXER WACHLER, MD, BOXER WACHLER VISION INSTITUTE

"Susan's wonderful and upbeat book, *Wired for High-Level Wellness*, shows us how we can all choose to be vibrantly healthy, happy, balanced, successful, peaceful, and heart-centered. She has taught me about all aspects of well-being, clean living, and how to maintain a healthy body, mind, and spirit in an everyday stressful life. In her book, Susan teaches us to see beauty and vitality in everyday living—even during stressful times—and to realize that age is just a number and we can choose to be youthful well into older age. If you simply want to enrich your experience of living, making your life a great adventure and celebration, then this esteemed book was written just for you. Susan even offers a couple of intermission breaks in the book with very humorous stories that had me laughing out loud. Not only does she provide a plethora of sound and practical health advice to help us all look and feel younger, boost energy, supercharge self-esteem, strengthen the brain, and cultivate an attitude of gratitude, but she also provides some delicious recipes that are easy and fast to get ready for busy people like me who want to eat healthfully and have limited time for meal preparation. I invite you to wake up to the fullness of life and all its potential, read *Wired for High-Level Wellness*, become informed and inspired, and live a healed life."

—MYRAN THOMAS, LA ESTHETIQUE WELLNESS

"*Wired for High-Level Wellness* is an important book for two reasons. First, it tells you that wellness is a choice. Second, it gives excellent advice on how to attain superb wellness once you've made the choice. Reading it will enable you to add to the vitality of the world."

—FINLEY W. BROWN, JR., MD

"I think everyone wants to be all they can be and live an inspired life. In her upbeat book *Wired for High-Level Wellness*, Susan Smith Jones gives us some valuable choices and easy-to-follow guidelines that can be used as building blocks in our lives that will allow us to be the best we can be. Creating a healthy, happy, peaceful, and balanced life is now well within our grasp, thanks to this empowering book."

—NANCY S. SCHORT, DDS

"Susan Smith Jones has been a favorite guest of mine on my health radio shows for over 15 years. Her enthusiasm, wealth of knowledge, and sense of humor shine through brightly in all of our radio discussions and my audiences always request her back soon. Even my production and recording team are delighted when she presents her healthy living topics. I first worked with Susan because of her wonderful books and work at UCLA as an expert in fitness and wellness. Susan is highly knowledgeable in holistic health and her books educate the public on how to achieve optimum health. In *Wired for High-Level Wellness*, she offers a beautiful and inspiring guide to living a life that is rooted in hope, faith, vitality, joy, and God's love. Reading about her Christian lifestyle and how her relationship with God is always at the center of her day-to-day activities will inspire and uplift you. When you read this book, you will feel like Susan is your friend, taking you by the hand and guiding you on your personal path to high-level wellness."

—KARLA CALUMET, PHD, HEALTH PSYCHOLOGIST

"Regardless of where you have looked for better health and how much 'dis-ease' you are experiencing now, you can begin to put it behind you by reading this book . . . and placing yourself on a path to enjoy the life you deserve. In *Wired for High-Level Wellness*, Susan provides practical yet powerful techniques, tips, and delicious recipes to help manage stress, support brain health, bolster immunity, increase self-esteem, restore well-being, and live a more peaceful, happy, and balanced life."

—ANGIE DUNKLING AVERILL, DMD, AND GORDON AVERILL, DMD,
26TH STREET DENTAL

"Dr. Susan has been a monthly guest on my radio program, *This Week in America*, for over 12 years. She is the only guest I've ever invited to participate monthly because she's a font of healthy living brilliance and has enthusiasm for every topic she discusses. In fact, Susan is one of the most amazing people I've ever known—a perfectly balanced person of inner strength, kindness, humor, and equanimity, and she's as smart as a whip. Susan is a gifted teacher who brings together modern research and ageless wisdom in all of her work and especially in her book *Wired for High-Level Wellness*. I've read many of Susan's books, and this one is my all-time favorite because it's a storehouse of life-altering holistic health knowledge and comprehension. I have one word of warning for you: Once you read this empowering, uplifting, and motivating book, you'll be inspired to make some major lifestyle changes for the better. Your IQ will go up, too! So get yourself ready, for a healthier and happier new you will emerge once you've met this glorious Renaissance lady through the pages of this electrifying book and incorporate her generous guidance into your day-to-day lifestyle."

—RIC BRATTON, FOUNDER, PRODUCER & HOST, *THIS WEEK IN AMERICA*

"At Hallelujah Diet, known for over two decades as Hallelujah Acres, we believe that food is medicine and that choosing to consume foods as close to the way God created them is the best diet to empower the self-healing God placed within each of us. When we follow His pattern, set forth in Genesis 1:29, we most often regain and sustain the level of health He designed us to enjoy. This means a whole-foods, plant-based diet rich in fresh vegetables and fruits. In *Wired for High-Level Wellness*, Susan shows us how these health-enriching foods can detoxify the body, support and improve brain function, keep us fit and trim, slow down the aging process, supercharge the immune system, and help us to look and feel our best well into older age. But this book is so much more than just sound nutritional advice and delicious, easy-to-prepare recipes. Susan also writes about her relationship with God and why it's the center of her life. She candidly reveals many personal challenges she has faced throughout her life and how she came out on the other side with more hope and faith, always determined to 'let go and let God.'

"Susan teaches that being vibrantly healthy is more than eating the best diet and jogging around the block a few times a week. She shows us that all of the countless choices we make every day reflect our level of self-esteem. Boosting our self-esteem is a central theme throughout *Wired for High-Level Wellness*. As she writes in the book's Introduction, 'In my own life, I fortify self-esteem through the principles of filling my life with vim and vigor, living a God-centered life, never letting anyone or anything cause me to doubt my ability to achieve my goals, staying committed to a healthy lifestyle, and always remembering that my body is God's temple and deserves to be treated lovingly—with respect and kindness.' The quality of our health is an integral part of our happiness. Susan gives us the tools we need to build solid health and, consequently, strengthen homes and families by passing along traditions that promote happy, healthful, and joyful lives. This inspiring book will enhance your life and keep on giving for years to come. Outstanding!"

—OLIN IDOL, ND, CNC, VICE PRESIDENT OF HEALTH, HALLELUJAH DIET

"Susan Smith Jones is the real thing. She's a walking, talking, living, breathing embodiment of what she gently preaches. For almost 30 years, Susan has been a regular guest on my many interview talk shows and has even filled in for me as host when I have been away. She always lights up the phone lines with her knowledge, enthusiasm, and humor, and I know that she will also light up your life with her healthy living books. All her beautifully designed books are filled with holistic health-enhancing information, and I've been captivated by all of them. But if I had to pick my favorite one, it would be *Wired for High-Level Wellness* because it has made such a profound difference in my life. As a result of her wisdom and guidance in this book, I lost all of my extra weight, upgraded my exercise program, healed my body, prospered in my life, feel more joyful, and am healthier and more energetic than ever. She has a unique ability to inspire and motivate in a way that makes you feel empowered and lets you know that your wellness destiny is under your control. My advice: get a copy of this book for yourself and then get several more copies to give as gifts to all your family and friends. Everyone will love it! And what better gift can you give than the gift of health?"

—NICK LAWRENCE, RADIO & TV TALK SHOW HOST/PRODUCER

"Incredibly practical and uplifting, *Wired for High-Level Wellness* shows simple and proven ways out of an unhealthy, stressful lifestyle—from what you eat, how you exercise, and what you think and feel—to a balanced life abounding with joy, vitality, and self-confidence. I especially appreciate Susan's personal stories and how she brings insight to life lessons we all need to learn in order to live our highest potential. Susan knows how to make her life and the lives of her clients and friends great adventures simply by making a commitment to live fully. You will learn how to do this in the pages of this book. *Wired for High-Level Wellness* is sure to be a welcome companion for anyone seeking to bring radiant health into their lives."

—Peter W. Brown, MD

"*Wired for High-Level Wellness* is a beautiful, clear, uplifting book. A guide to living healthfully, joyfully, and peacefully, it is also a fine example of the God- and faith-centeredness that bring grace to life. As Susan writes about in her preface, the Bible is her favorite book that she consults every day, and she features many of her favorite Bible quotes throughout the pages of this life-enriching book. If you are ready to improve your diet, reduce stress in your life, exercise your way to vibrant health, increase your self-esteem, achieve your heartfelt goals, feel more hopeful and positive, and develop a closer relationship with God, *Wired for High-Level Wellness* is the book for you; it's loaded with secrets to improve the quality of your life."

—Pastor Brittian Bowman

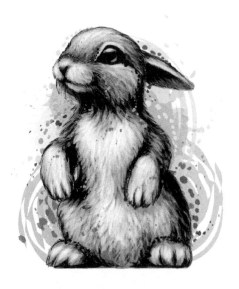

Wired for High-Level WELLNESS

Simple Ways to Rejuvenate, Meditate & Prosper

SUSAN SMITH JONES, PHD

Foreword by David Craddock, MA

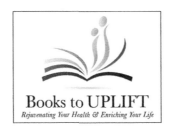

Books to UPLIFT
Rejuvenating Your Health & Enriching Your Life

The health suggestions and recommendations in this book are based on the training, research, and personal experiences of the author. Because each person and each situation is unique, the author and publisher encourage the reader to check with his or her physician or other health professional before using any procedure outlined in this book. Neither the author nor the publisher is responsible for any adverse consequences resulting from any of the suggestions in this book.

Published by Books to UPLIFT
Los Angeles, CA

ISBN: 978-0-9991492-7-0

Copyright © by Susan Smith Jones, PhD

All Rights Reserved. No part of this book may be reproduced or transmitted in any form or by any means, electronic or mechanical, including photocopying, or by any information storage and retrieval system, except for the purpose of brief excerpts for articles, books, or reviews, without the written permission of the author.

Cover and interior design: Gary A. Rosenberg

For further information and permission approval, contact: Health Unlimited, PO Box 49215, Los Angeles, CA 90049, Attn. Manager

Printed in the United States of America.

Also by Susan Smith Jones, PhD

Please refer to **SusanSmithJones.com** to learn more about
these and her other books or to purchase any of them.

Invest in Yourself with Exercise

The Curative Kitchen & Lifestyle

Be the Change

Kitchen Gardening:
Rejuvenate with Homegrown Sprouts

Vegetable Soup/The Fruit Bowl
(with Dianne Warren, for children ages 1-10)

Choose to Thrive

A Hug in a Mug: Using Herbal Teas,
Culinary Spices & Fresh Juices as Medicine

UPLIFTED 12 Minutes to More Joy,
Faith, Peace, Kindness & Vitality

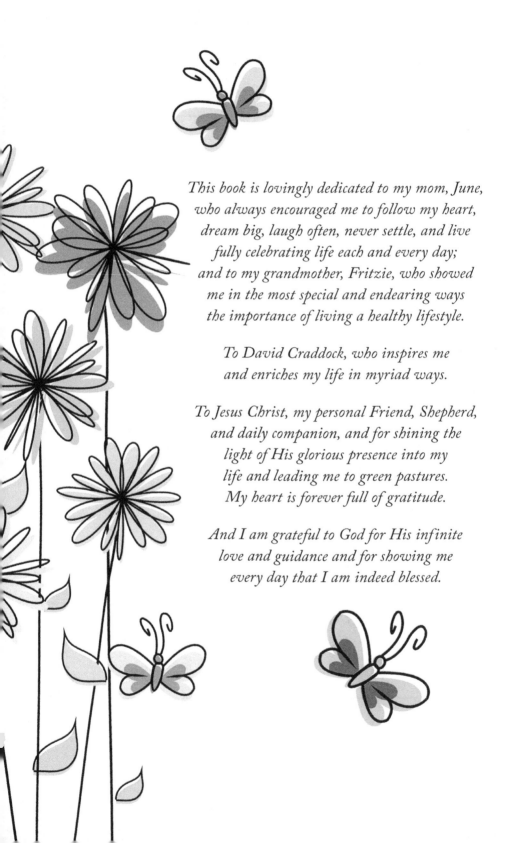

This book is lovingly dedicated to my mom, June,
who always encouraged me to follow my heart,
dream big, laugh often, never settle, and live
fully celebrating life each and every day;
and to my grandmother, Fritzie, who showed
me in the most special and endearing ways
the importance of living a healthy lifestyle.

To David Craddock, who inspires me
and enriches my life in myriad ways.

To Jesus Christ, my personal Friend, Shepherd,
and daily companion, and for shining the
light of His glorious presence into my
life and leading me to green pastures.
My heart is forever full of gratitude.

And I am grateful to God for His infinite
love and guidance and for showing me
every day that I am indeed blessed.

PSALM 23
A Psalm of David (RSV)

1 The Lord is my shepherd, I shall not want; **2** He makes me lie down in green pastures. He leads me beside still waters; **3** He restores my soul. He leads me in paths of righteousness for his name's sake. **4** Even though I walk through the valley of the shadow of death, I fear no evil; for thou art with me; thy rod and thy staff, they comfort me. **5** Thou preparest a table before me in the presence of my enemies; thou anointest my head with oil, my cup overflows. **6** Surely goodness and mercy shall follow me all the days of my life; and I shall dwell in the house of the Lord forever.

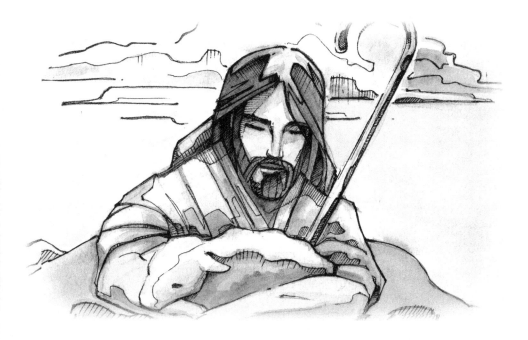

It doesn't matter if a million people tell you what you can't do, or if ten million people tell you no. If you get one YES from God, that's ALL you need.

~TYLER PERRY

Have faith that nothing is impossible. I trust that all of the unexpected changes in my daily and weekly schedule are a result of God making the necessary adjustments to help my days and life unfold in Divine Order.

~SUSAN SMITH JONES (FROM *BE THE CHANGE*)

The secret to learning well is: eat half, walk double, laugh triple, and love without measure.

~TIBETAN PROVERB

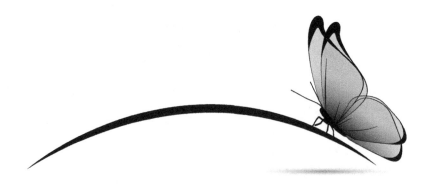

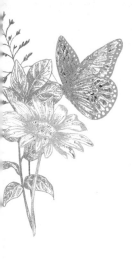

Contents

Susan's Favorites

*Take delight in the Lord, and He will
give you the desires of your heart.*

~Psalm 37:4

*To laugh often and much; to win the respect of intelligent
people and the affection of children; to earn the appreciation
of honest critics and endure the betrayal of false friends; to
appreciate beauty; to find the best in others; to leave the world
a bit better, whether by a healthy child, a garden patch, or a
redeemed social condition; to know even one life has breathed
easier because you have lived. This is to have succeeded.*

~Ralph Waldo Emerson

*As human beings, our job in life is to help people realize
how rare and valuable each one of us really is, that each
of us has something that no one else has—or ever will
have-something inside that is unique to all time.*

~Fred Rogers

*My child, do not forget my teaching, but keep my
commands in your heart, for they will prolong your life
many years and bring you peace and prosperity.*

~Proverbs 3:1-2

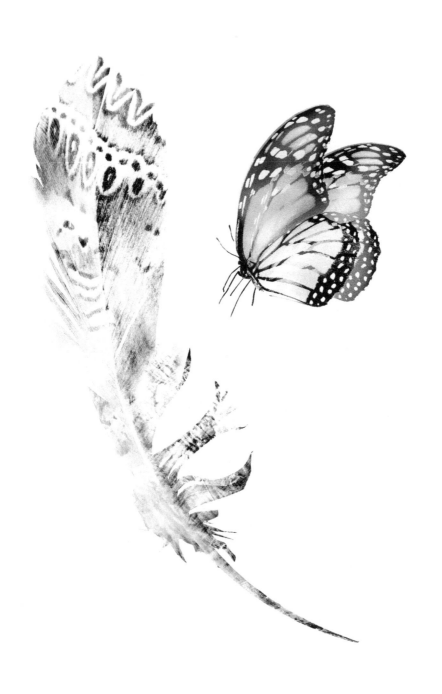

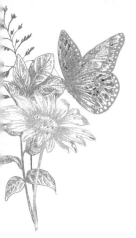

Foreword

Be yourself—everyone else is already taken.

~Oscar Wilde

*38 For I am convinced that neither death nor life,
neither angels nor demons, neither the present nor the
future, nor any powers, 39 neither height nor depth, nor
anything else in all creation, will be able to separate us
from the love of God that is in Christ Jesus our Lord.*

~Romans 8:38-39

Once upon a time, there was a sweet baby girl born in Los Angeles the last day of November to happy parents and grandparents. Her childhood was filled with books to read, daily outdoor activity frolicking barefoot on the grass or the sand at the beach in Santa Monica, and family outings around the country with her mom and siblings. Her name was Susan and little did she know at the time, but her career in holistic health and writing was taking root and being fertilized.

In Susan's teen years and twenties, as you will read in the introduction to this book, she faced several serious challenges that further shaped and stimulated her career. These trails taught her deep in her core how essential it is to always put your faith and reliance on God, how with enough faith we can move mountains, why we must always keep hope and determination alive, and how the glorious human body can be healed and revitalized through a consistent healthy living program.

In her teens, Susan's maternal grandmother, Fritzie, who came from Denmark to America through Ellis Island, taught her about the importance of eating foods close to the way nature made them, making fresh juice and green smoothies, growing sprouts in the kitchen, and living a healthy lifestyle. Fritzie also encouraged Susan to get the best education possible (which she did—obtaining several degrees from the University of California, Los Angeles—UCLA) and to hone her speaking skills so she could inspire others with her understanding, wit, and wisdom.

Just as Susan and her mom were very close throughout their lives together, Susan and Fritzie were also devoted to each other's well-being. But it was Fritzie who taught her, starting in her early childhood years, about the wisdom of the Bible—the word of God—and about the teachings of Jesus.

From a very young age, Susan always felt a powerful and comforting relationship with Jesus, as she writes about in the Preface, as she always feels His Presence inside her in her daily life. When other friends had imaginary companions, Susan always had Jesus with her—and it's still the same for her to this day.

Susan's career took off and she fulfilled her mom's and grandmother's dreams for her traveling the world promoting her healthful living books, undertaking keynote addresses, lectures, workshops, and participating in media interviews on television and radio and for newspapers.

That's how I first met Susan, and it was just at the right time because my health was at an all-time low. I was 80 pounds overweight, stressed to the max with work, had irritating allergies for over 30 years, and was told by a doctor that if I didn't start making my health a priority, I would not be long for this world.

I believed that keeping our body temple vibrant and robust was essential, but I did not know where to start. Almost 12 years ago, as providence would have it, God brought this remarkable lady, Susan, to London, England, near where I lived, to give three motivating and life-enriching talks about healthy living that were exactly what I needed to hear. In previous years, I had heard other speakers discuss a variety of health topics, but no one ever inspired or empowered me like Susan's did.

This kind-to-a-fault, blue-eyed, blond-haired, shining example of God's vibrant health has an uncanny ability to take complex ideas and research and distill them into easy-to-understand, life-changing information and practical guidance. I also appreciate how she weaves into her books and talks her love of God and Jesus. It was no surprise that at the end of all three of her presentations to hundreds of people, Susan got vigorous standing ovations.

When her final talk was over on the last day in late June, I mustered up the courage to ask Susan to meet with me privately in the lecture hall in the hopes that she could help me personally with my many health issues. I reckoned that the worst thing that could happen is that she wouldn't have time to visit with me, but it was worth a try. Lucky for me, she agreed and that first hour-long encounter was one of the richest blessings in my life. Susan was patient, thoughtful, a great listener, attentive to all I was saying, very funny, and ever so perspicacious.

After our visit, Susan invited my mum and me to come to Santa Monica near her home the following December into early January for a private holistic health retreat just for us for two weeks. The transformations my mum and I made in our health and fitness was nothing short of a miracle. If you want to read about the detailed holistic program she put us both on during those memorable fourteen days and our amazing achievements, please refer to the forewords I wrote for her books *Invest in Yourself with Exercise* and *Choose to Thrive*.

Susan's books, website, and work have blessed the lives of millions of people around the globe and probably no one more than me. Her teachings and guidance helped me lose over 80 pounds, healed my annoying allergies, bolstered my energy, made me fit and strong, helped me achieve my career goals, and so much more. Susan even set up a personal gym for me in my home, upgraded my sartorial elegance, and did a makeover of my home's exterior design to spruce it up and improved my garden landscapes in both my front and back yards. Susan is a Renaissance woman and her attitude is that, with God, everything is possible; I haven't found anything yet that she doesn't do well. She often reminds me that her inner counsel with Jesus helps her with everything she thinks, feels, says, and does.

Since I now have a home in Los Angeles as well as in England, I have the pleasure of visiting often with Susan, and with each visit, I am inspired to take my wellness to a higher level thanks to her encouragement and sagacious, salubrious recommendations. This is something for which I thank God every day, for bringing Susan into my life.

Over meals, during hikes, long walks on the beach, or driving, we talk about God, Jesus, and our purpose in the world. We often fine-tune my healthy living program and make new goals I want to achieve to reach the highest level of wellness possible.

At this point, you might be wondering how I was so blessed to write the foreword for this book. Well, it was about eighteen months ago and Susan was in England giving many talks throughout the UK for churches, community groups, and a couple corporations. She was also participating in interviews on the BBC and other talk shows discussing simple ways we can all achieve high-level wellness no matter where our level of health is at present moment or how much we have sabotaged our health in the past.

During her media tour, I marveled at her keen mind, her ability to discuss just about anything with savvy, and her quick-witted humor when she talked about brain health, superfoods, a courageous and balanced life, God-connecting meditation, and oil pulling. On a few occasions, she also showed people how to make healthy meals and discussed why we need to keep stress levels down, the importance of being more childlike, embracing silence and solitude, the benefits of infrared saunas (or heat therapy), molecular hydrogen remedies, alkaline water, earthing or grounding, and having the courage to dream BIG and never let anyone or anything cause us to doubt our ability to achieve our goals. She even had discussions on prosperity and how to get in the flow of God's abundance that's readily available to us all 24/7. It was fascinating to watch her in action and the countless questions delivered her way to obtain her advice and suggestions on all of these topics. That's something about Susan I know well; she is rarely at a loss for words.

Whether with small or large audiences, in person, or during TV or radio interviews, her enthusiasm for high-level wellness, and life in general, is contagious, and it was easy to see that everyone who experienced Susan's unique blend of ancient wisdom, modern science, and common-sense approach to healthy living was as inspired and incentivized as I was. She is very easygoing and so enjoyable to be around. Everyone can feel that in her presence. When you are talking to her, you feel like you are friends and you have her full attention. How very rare that is these days when so many people are not fully engaged with you when you are talking to them. You can tell their mind is somewhere else. Without a doubt, with Susan, you feel appreciated, valued, and acknowledged for your blessing in her life at that moment. It's a joy to behold!

I accompanied her on her *Wired for High-Level Wellness* media tour throughout the United Kingdom, partly because of the educational experience it afforded me to learn as much as possible about all aspects of healing the body and creating radiant health, and also because she makes me laugh a lot and I love being in her presence. People came from all over the UK and other counties to hear her speak.

In many of the talks, she would begin with asking what countries people came from to see who traveled the farthest. In one of these talks in which I was contributing to the discussion of living a healthy life-style, and I was standing upfront with her, someone asked what country Susan is from thinking she had an accent (which she did to all of these people), so I jumped in with a quick response on the whiteboard. I wrote SUSAN and separated the letters a tad and told everyone, "Here's an easy way to remember where Susan is from." I pointed to the "S" and said "Susan," then pointed to the "USA" and said, "she is from the United States of America," and finally I pointed to the "N" and said the word "Noble." "So you see, Susan's an American Noble," I boasted because of my spontaneous creativity, which made Susan smile and blush and the audience laugh. And the truth is, she is very much a noble lady from the USA.

When Susan's tour was over, we carved out time to take a half-day hike (four hours!) in the beautiful, scenic hills of Staffordshire located in central England. During this quite arduous hike up and down very steep hills, we would constantly compete with one another to see who could make it to the top of the hill the fastest. Our competitive natures blend well, and we always push each other to achieve our best times and ever-greater accomplishments.

During this hike, we even managed to talk when the path was more level or took us downhill. Thinking about all of the myriad topics she had covered the previous couple of weeks during her media tour, I thought to myself, *Wouldn't it be terrific if she would put all of this material into the form of a book so I could have it on hand to go over often and also to gift others with this book.* So when we had a chance to stop briefly to drink some water and eat a banana, I broached the topic with her and said, "Susan, everywhere you went, people were so receptive and open to your eclectic discussions on wellness and always seemed to want more. Why don't you write a book with the same title of *Wired for High-Level Wellness* with an emphasis on how to rejuvenate the body head-to-toe, and include ways to commune with God through meditation and how we can all be a magnet for God's riches in our lives? Oh yes, and also incorporate some of your simple and delicious recipes for the green smoothies you are always making for us." And then I added this: "Since I am no longer a young man in my biological age (Susan has taught me that my age is only a number and that we are all as young as we feel, and I feel very youthful), I'd also like to request that you add in a chapter or two about brain health, as you talked about in the corporate lectures and on the television shows, and how to keep the brain sharp and focused; tell us all how to keep our brain cells and all of our faculties intact and in the pink well into older age. I know that many of my friends and business associates would also appreciate learning more about this significant topic."

Well, I am pleased to say that my suggestion of a new book stopped her in her tracks and she was so overjoyed with excitement and enthusiasm that she all of a sudden did a cartwheel on the apex of a very steep hill. That's another characteristic about Susan: She is always surprising you with what she says and does and her rich enthusiasm for enjoying life shines through in all of her quotidian pursuits and activities.

And then she said to me with a somewhat quizzical expression on her face, "I'll tell you what—let's race to the next hill's apex and there I will give you my answer to your request of me," and off she went getting a head start on me, as she often does. I must have stimulated her brain and got her enthusiasm bubbling over because I could not catch up to her on this fast trek. When I finally reached her with our usual "high five" congratulatory tap at our accomplishment, with her usually beaming smile, she told me she loved my book idea and would make it happen, but only with the condition that I write the foreword, again, for this book. Truth be told, she didn't have to twist my arm at all to encourage me to say yes to her offer. It is always my pleasure and blessing to write forewords for any of her outstanding and life-enhancing books.

All the way back down, and until the end of this four-hour-hike, we couldn't stop talking about the contents of this book. By the time we finished the hike, we were both energized mentally from all of our discussions, inspired spiritually from God's bountiful nature all around us for hours of hiking and respites of prayer time, and physically satisfied from the challenging, gradient hill workout and accomplishment of finishing the course in our best time ever!

Next, we were meeting a couple friends for lunch at a café nearby the hike's trailhead, and we both mentioned how hungry we were for a healthy meal, which we definitely earned from the trek that started early morning. We arrived first at the café and agreed equally that sitting down was most welcomed. As we were savoring a couple glasses each of room temperature lemon water, our friends arrived and joined us saying as they sat down, "We are exhausted because there was no parking available in front of the café and we just had to walk two agonizing blocks to get here." Our friend said he was going to ask his wife to get the car after lunch so he didn't have to walk so far again. Susan and I quickly smiled at each other and tapped our knees under the table.

We both intuitively knew that we'd keep quiet about our multi-hour hike on steep terrain so as not to make this couple feel embarrassed or uncomfortable.

However, we did take this opportunity to talk to them about this new book idea that I gave to Susan and we asked them what information would appeal to them to include. Since they were both often stressed out in their careers, they suggested info on how to keep the body and mind calm when challenges and difficulties rear their ugly heads in life. They wanted to learn about meditation, what it really means, how to do it, and how to reap the benefits. They also wanted to learn more about our Christian lifestyles in the book as a way to inspire them to strengthen their relationships with God and Jesus, and why the Bible is so important to Susan and me. Since Susan often speaks about the healing power of living with gratitude every day, our friends wanted to read more on this topic in the book.

After our friends left, Susan and I stayed at the café to talk some more about the contents of this book and to create the outline. Being positive and optimistic is Susan's normal way of being, and when we are together, we have a grand time discussing anything and everything on creating our very best lives. Hours fly by when we are engrossed in mind-stimulating and health-enhancing topics. And I am often gobsmacked at her magnificently positive and infectious enthusiasm to everyday situations and all life.

When others hear how well I know Susan, I am often asked to describe her characteristics, hobbies, and interests. That's quite easy for me to do. More than anything, she loves to be out in nature where she feels ever so close to God, Jesus, and her angels. She has a close relationship with her guardian angels and talks to me about this often. In fact, they are ever so close to Susan and help her with achieving her goals and dreams, appreciating life's simple blessings, seeing the best in others, and orchestrating the minutiae of her daily life. She is, indeed, a very caring and ebullient person, always seeking to look for the best in everyone and everything.

Laughter is an elixir for her, and she laughs often and is also a practical joker, as I've written about in the foreword for her book *Be the Change*, but never in a way that would hurt or humiliate another person. Susan frequently puts coins in peoples' parking meters so they don't get tickets. She goes out of her way to show kindness to others. It was her mom who taught her about the importance of living by the Golden Rule, which is the main tenet by which she lives each day. In fact, there's never been a time when she was driving us somewhere in the USA or in England that she didn't let in another driver when requested or thank other drivers for letting us in. It's just her nature to be kindhearted and good-natured, and she has taught me so much about the value of kindness and living by the Golden Rule from Matthew 7:12 ("Do unto others as you would have them do unto you").

Susan is, indeed, a wordsmith and is often carrying around a dictionary to study. I've never seen anyone else do this, and in Chapter 1, you will understand why she is a true logophile. Susan is especially fond of words that end in "ful." So if I needed to describe Susan with only "ful" words—something she will greatly appreciate when she reads this foreword, here's what I would say. Susan is . . .

Blissful	*Playful*	*Skillful*	*Truthful*	*Merciful*
Youthful	*Resourceful*	*Peaceful*	*Gleeful*	*Beautiful*
Zestful	*Dutiful*	*Masterful*		

. . . and just plain *WONDERFUL!*

Susan loves to do media work on television and radio talk shows to discuss any health- and life-enriching topic, and she favors any discussion about living a God-centered life. She's told me before, "If I can inspire people to take better care of their bodies and health, and also develop a closer relationship to God, then I will have fulfilled the purpose God has bestowed on me."

More specifically, in keeping with Susan's Christian faith, most of her favorite TV and radio shows in which to participate are the Christian programs because she is free to not only talk about holistic health, often lacking on most of these TV programs, but most especially about her very close and personal relationship with God and Jesus.

What she loves the most, which also is wonderful for me, too, is when we do Christian TV shows together. As a devout Christian myself, I know the entire Bible well from decades of personal study and preparations for my countless talks for churches, schools, and community groups about Christian lifestyle matters and living a balanced, peaceful, and God-focused life. "With your wealth of knowledge on the Bible, and my comprehension of holistic health, my preference is to visit talk shows together so we can offer the most well-rounded, uplifting discussions," Susan has mentioned to me on many occasions. "From Susan's mouth to God's ears," I affirm aloud and silently.

I am confident you will also derive tremendous value from this masterful and eclectic compendium, *Wired for High-Level Wellness*. Susan reminds us that we were created by God and have been blessed with a miraculous body. From head to toe, she shows us how to not only heal the body but also create robust health . . . at any age. We were not created to simply get by with an unrewarding, unfulfilling, and prosaic life. God wants each of us to flourish, thrive, and live our best life. It's difficult to do this if we are dealing with health issues—big or small.

As you put Susan's key principles and suggestions into action, you will quickly feel the difference and start glowing with vitality. Her easy-to-follow program is an indispensable and refreshing change from most health and self-improvement books that only focus on one particular aspect of health. Balance is the key, and Susan will keep you focused on the long-term results that come from choosing a healthy lifestyle. No matter your reason for turning to this book—whether it's to find more happiness in life, look and feel better, find balance, discover how to eat healthier and be more positive, reinvigorate your body, boost your self-esteem, and/or live a more peaceful, hopeful, prosperous life with a heart full of faith and a strengthened relationship with God—this book will lead you in the right direction. Get ready to feel wonderful in body, mind, and spirit and enjoy the extraordinary life you were designed to live.

—David Craddock
DavidCraddock.com

Do not pray for an easy life,
pray for the strength to endure.

~BRUCE LEE

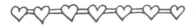

4 Love is patient, love is kind. It does not envy, it does
not boast, it is not proud. 5 It does not dishonor others,
it is not self-seeking, it is not easily angered, it keeps no
record of wrongs. 6 Love does not delight in evil but
rejoices with the truth. 7 It always protects, always trusts,
always hopes, always perseveres. 8 Love never fails.

~1 CORINTHIANS 13:4-8

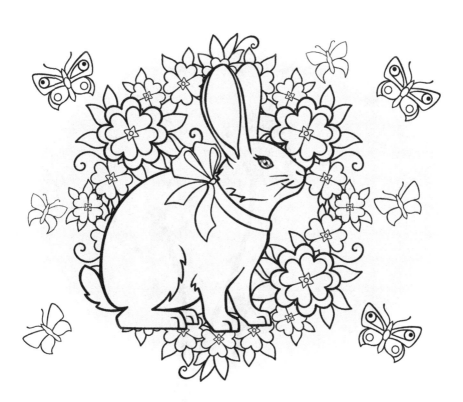

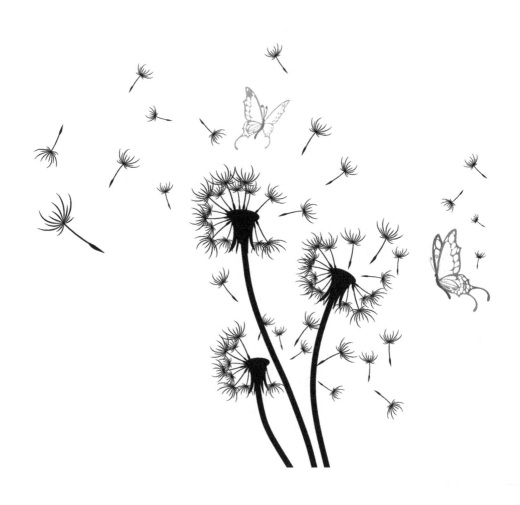

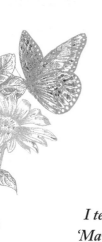

Preface

I tell you the truth, you can say to this mountain,
'May you be lifted up and thrown into the sea,' and
it will happen. But you must really believe it will
happen and have no doubt in your heart.

~MARK 11:23

You already have within you the excellent power of God;
you just need to stir it up and release it.

~2 CORINTHIANS 4:7

When I was a little girl, my grandmother, Fritzie, would talk to me about the love that Jesus Christ had for me and how He would live inside me as my companion and personal friend for the rest of my life, my guiding light, and the source of inner wisdom and empowerment in my life. She was right and when I was a preteen, in choosing to trust in Jesus, I began my lifelong experience of feeling His love and presence in my life. I would talk to Him often and ask for guidance and always have the assurance of His understanding. As I grew older and became a teenager, Fritzie would often read the Bible to me telling me frequently that the Bible is the word of God that would bring me close to God. She encouraged me to read the Bible every day, even if only for a couple minutes, which I still do to this day. I write about Fritzie's positive influence in my Christian lifestyle and our close relationship in my books *Be the Change* and *Kitchen Gardening*.

Now as an adult, I continue to strengthen my Christian lifestyle by choosing to live a God-centered life. Putting God first in my life is the hub of the wheel for me and all else takes a backseat to my relationship with Jesus. I have many Bibles in my home and even keep one in my car for ongoing reference during the day. I take one with me when I travel in the United States and overseas and enjoy looking at the many different translations for passages, a practice that enhances my understanding about what each passage is seeking to teach me. Because of my reverence for the Bible, you will find many different Bible quotes in this book. Most of them you might already be familiar with and others may be new to you.

For me, the glorious work that we call the Bible is so much more than copious amounts of text in books, chapters, and verses. It's a beautiful compilation of ancient wisdom, inspired by God, in the form of letters, poems, and moving stories that have transformed the way I feel and think about my life and life in general. Every page has something special and meaningful for each one of us. It even has romantic stories and life-enriching passages that teach us about the most important aspects of life—from heartfelt love, to relationships, to faith, to right action and thought, to achieving our goals and realizing our dreams. It has *Everything* we need to teach us how to thrive and flourish in our lives. If you haven't picked up the Bible in months, years, or decades, do it soon. It will profoundly change your life for the better. Oftentimes, before I engage in my morning and evening prayer time and meditation, I will open up the Bible at random and see what message that page has for me. Wherever I open, it's always relevant in my life and that gives me the assurance that God is with me and guiding me every day.

The Bible truly is a masterpiece inspired from heaven, best understood by recognizing that the Old Testament and the New Testament are one coherent whole, with the New Testament as the fulfillment of the Old Testament. How deeply grateful we are to the Jewish people who took enormous care to chronicle all the events that we read about in Holy Scripture and what a privilege it is to have this testimony of timeless wisdom preserved for us over the generations! The contribution of the Jewish tradition to our Biblical understanding, when viewed through the prism of the life and ministry, death and resurrection of Jesus, is a wonder to behold. The New Testament is then the record of all the love and truth that was and continues to this day to be released into this world by Jesus in all His power and presence as expressed in the lives of His followers, those who have chosen to respond to His message.

Throughout the pages of this book, you will find I refer to the Holy Spirit, God, Heavenly Father, Jesus as Lord or Savior or both, Jesus as the Christ, God and Jesus as the Divine, and other terms that resonate in my heart. In your own Bible study, you will find other terminology that describes God and Jesus. Whichever words I use on various pages, my hope is that you will feel my devotion to the one true God, as Dear Lord and Heavenly Father who wants to give good gifts to His children.

As mentioned a few different ways in this book, I believe that God has provided us with the gift of an amazing body that is truly a miracle of miracles. Treating our body disrespectfully by eating an unhealthy diet, living a sedentary life, being pessimistic about daily circumstances, or feeling powerless to make positive changes in our life is not what God intended. We are one with God, co-creators with the Divine and nothing is impossible. We can achieve our goals and live magnificent lives. Being vibrant and healthy and taking care of your body is a very good place to start, since the body reflects the mind, and the mind reflects the spirit. We are body, mind, and spirit working as one. So one of our gifts back to our Heavenly Father is to simply take loving care of our body.

> *Living an uncluttered life gives me time for things I really care about, like time to think, to read, to walk in nature, to take loving care of my body, to meditate and commune with God, and to watch the sunrise or sunset.*
>
> ~SUSAN SMITH JONES

Each day is another opportunity to strengthen our relationship with God and to see the Divine in everyone and everything. My wish and aspiration day in, day out is to make each day a love note and prayer to God by how I choose to live. As it says in the Bible in **1 Thessalonians 5:17,** *Pray without ceasing.*

The goal of this book is to teach you how to take the best care of your body, mind, and spirit. High-level wellness is within our grasp if we choose it each day. Our body temple houses the spirit of God so making a commitment to love, respect, and honor your God-given body is one of the most important commitments you can make.

Always remember that the Bible has all of the answers to the questions for which you are seeking guidance. Choose today to be inspired by all of its wisdom.

You might enjoy my Christian website David Craddock and I created together. Here you will learn more about how I am uplifted and inspired by the Bible and more.

ChristianLifestyleMatters.com

For with God, nothing will be impossible.

~LUKE 1:37

Peace I leave with you, my peace I give to you; not as the world gives do I give to you. Let not your heart be troubled, neither let it be afraid.

~JOHN 14:27

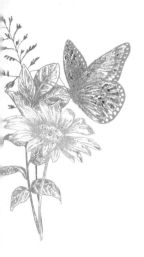

Introduction

There is a blessing in the air.

~WILLIAM WORDSWORTH

*Do not go where the path may lead. Go instead
where there is no path and leave a trail.*

~RALPH WALDO EMERSON

*I*f you've picked up this book, chances are that you are seeking change in your life—not just a new hairstyle or a fresh wardrobe, but lasting, meaningful, and resounding change for your sense of health and happiness.

You have definitely come to the right place! *Wired for High-Level Wellness* is a compendium of wisdom and practical suggestions that reveal how to create a life of robust self-esteem, vibrant physical health from head-to-toe, powerful prosperity, and a deepened connection with God. I even include green smoothie recipes and a few other delicious, nutritious recipes in Chapter 17. The wisdom and practicable common sense in the book is culled from over 35 years of experience as an educator, consultant, and motivational speaker in the fields of holistic health and human potential. But I haven't just *studied* how to make lasting change in your life—I've lived it since I was a teenager! And, for me, the catalysts of change in my life have often arrived in packages I was not expecting.

We've all heard the clichés: "Change begins with you" or "Change begins with choice." While it's true that authentic transformation comes from within and modifying your life necessitates a deliberate commitment to new thoughts and behaviors, sometimes the catalysts of change are delivered from external sources. That has definitely been the case in my life. As you embark on your journey of change and upgrading your life, using this book as your companion, I'd like to first share some of my life-altering experiences to offer hope and guidance to light your path, which I shared only briefly in one of my previous books entitled *Kitchen Gardening*.

The Mind/Body/Spirit Connection

When I was barely 17, my father unexpectedly passed away. I was devastated. I had no precedent for this type of deep loss and no skills to cope with it. My way of dealing with the tragedy was by, really, not dealing with it at all. I stuffed all my feelings inside and numbed myself with food—typical teenage temptations of fast-food burgers, pizza, and sugary sweets and pastries galore. Today, I would recognize this binging behavior as a hallmark of depression, but back then I didn't realize what was going on. After a year of managing my grief by eating everything in sight, my health took a nosedive. I developed allergies, asthma, acne, and joint pain, not to mention I had gained a considerable amount of weight.

While I suffered physically, the emotional toll was even greater. Before my father's death, I had been an active and social teenager. Now an overweight high school student with acne, I became the subject of jokes around campus and was bullied by people I thought were my friends. I was rapidly losing any semblance of confidence and self-esteem. My heart was heavy, and I was sinking emotionally. Pain was devouring my will to live. It was not a pretty picture.

Luckily for me, there was another catalyst of change already present in my life: my beloved grandmother, whom I called Fritzie. Like many grandmothers, Fritzie was kind, nurturing, and full of wisdom, but she also possessed a vast wealth of knowledge about holistic health and the human body. When she saw my physical and emotional state a year after my father's passing, she knew immediately that I needed healing from the inside out.

Her first step was to take me to our family doctor for a checkup to make sure there was no life-threatening disease that had taken hold. When I told the doctor my symptoms, he apprised me that I would have to live with my newly developed allergies, asthma, joint pain, and acne the rest of my life because, as he said, "It was in my genes." Leaving his office with a handful of prescriptions that he implored us to fill immediately, I felt even more depressed and powerless. Clearly, he was a very unevolved and ignorant doctor with no concept of how the body can heal itself if we give it all of the very best ingredients from nature and live a healthful lifestyle.

My grandmother, in all her wisdom, instead took me home and had a heart-to-heart talk with me. She told me that if I followed her suggestions 100%, my health issues and depression would disappear within 30 days. She said my acne would clear up, my asthma would dissipate, my energy would soar, the extra weight I gained would melt away, and my attitude would change from negative and powerless to positive and hopeful.

Needless to say, she had my attention. A wise person once said, "When the student is ready, the teacher will appear," and this was definitely true for me. I was ready.

Fritzie started by overhauling my diet of processed snack foods and sweets. She was an advocate of eating foods as close to the way nature made them as possible. "In nature," she firmly reminded me often, "we won't find ice cream trees, potato chip bushes, or doughnut vines." Though I initially resisted eating the colorful vegetables, fresh juices, green smoothies, nutrient-rich sprouts, and other living foods she prepared for me (what teenager wouldn't?!), soon enough I became a believer. The pounds started coming off, my skin became clear and vibrant again, my asthma was soothed, my joints were pain-free, and my outlook improved.

Fritzie also went to work on healing my spirit. A devout Christian, as you now know that I am also, she knew that the problem underlying my poor diet and physical ailments was the loss of my father. I would often hear her say, "The body reflects the mind and the mind reflects the spirit." She explained to me that even when our lives are burdened with loss and tragedy, we can still find much for which to be grateful. One of the first things she taught me was to begin each day talking to Jesus/God and then blessing everything—blessing the sunrise, the happy sounds of the morning birds singing their song, my unlimited opportunities, my potential to create whatever I wanted, and anything I had planned for the day already.

Whether I was with Fritzie or alone, I would always start each day with prayer, reading the Bible, and spending a few moments in communion with God. It always lifted my mood and made me feel gloriously hopeful and optimistic—even to this day.

Fritzie said that beginning the day on a positive note would set the tone for the entire day. She was right about making each morning a positive experience—and also about *everything!*

She would often ask me to tell her some of my favorite Bible quotes, which I have sprinkled throughout the pages of this book. I liked to please her and learning many Bible quotes was a joy for me and helped me get through each day keeping my strong connection to God. The wisdom of countless Bible quotes, when we keep them readily available in the forefront of our brains, can help us all navigate through the challenges and sometimes difficult tasks of everyday living. One of the many favorites of both of ours is . . .

If you do not stand firm in your faith,
you will not stand at all.
~Isaiah 7:9

Fritzie always reminded me to cultivate and choose an attitude of gratitude (and you'll read about this more in Part 5), which included speaking only positive words and affirmations, even when appearances showed me the opposite. Her voice is ingrained in my mind saying, "Attitude is the mind's paintbrush; it can color anything." She suggested that I recite these three affirmations daily: "I behold the Divine (God) in everyone and everything," "Only the best for me," and "With Christ as my daily companion, nothing is impossible." I was surprised by how approaching each day from a perspective of hope and gratitude began to assuage my grief for my father. I started to see the world as an inviting, abundant place once again.

At the end of the 30 days, an astounding transformation occurred. Not only had transformative changes in my health, appearance, and attitude taken place, but the tools for lasting change had taken root and were wired internally within me. I was becoming wired for high-level wellness and vitality. It was truly an inside job and started with my attitude and perspective.

With all her wisdom and down-to-earth common sense, Fritzie had enlightened me to the benefits of taking care of my body from head to toe, inside and out. I learned to listen to my body's whisperings and look to God's bounty of natural remedies. It felt like a new and glorious way to live—in God's hands with nature's treasure trove as my partner. Needless to say, I threw the doctor's prescriptions away.

In this book, I hope to be a catalyst of change for you, just as Fritzie was a catalyst of change for me. Though the wealth of information in *Wired for High-Level Wellness* has been selected from many years of study and my experience working with thousands of people around the world, Fritzie's (along with June's—my mom) commonsense teachings are its foundations. Ultimately, change must come from inside you, but that doesn't mean you don't need the loving hand of a knowledgeable guide to start you down the path. Through this book, I am taking your hand in mine and guiding you on the road to victory. It's yours for the choosing. Make the commitment and ask God to brightly light your path.

A Leap of Faith

In the years after I recovered from grieving for my father, I felt as if I could conquer any problem that came my way and that my vibrant health was foolproof. I kept a diet loaded with fresh fruits and vegetables, an active lifestyle (I loved baseball and once dreamed of being the first female Los Angeles Dodgers player!), and an outlook of gratitude and positivity. As long as I continued to tend to my mind, my body, and my spirit, I felt that I was invincible.

But of course, the Universe is never static, and change came knocking on my door once again. I had to open another unwelcome package.

In my twenties, I was in a terrible automobile accident. Though I felt lucky to have lived, I fractured my back so badly that doctors told me I would never again be physically active and would live a life of chronic pain. I plunged into despair because all of a sudden my life and my body no longer felt like they were in my control.

While Fritzie's tactics had easily helped me shed pounds and regain balance as a teenager, I knew they wouldn't be enough to heal a fractured back. Something was telling me that I would need even stronger tools. I knew I couldn't sidestep my sadness and struggle. I needed to face my difficulties head-on. I love these words from David Wolpe, Rabbi of Sinai Temple in Los Angeles, who said the following: "The measure of human character is our reaction to dark times. No one can sidestep darkness. It is the throne upon which light sits. If a soul has not known sadness and struggle, there is no chance of overcoming, no cherishing the dawn."

Searching for answers, I sat in silence one evening on a bench at sunset, gazing at the ocean near my home in West Los Angeles, California, on the bluff overlooking the Santa Monica Bay. Suddenly, I had an epiphany. As always, I felt Jesus next to me on the bench and God's loving presence and knew that His plan for me wasn't a life of pain. All at once, I realized the missing tool that I needed was *faith*. In all his sagacity, it was Ralph Waldo Emerson who wrote this soul-stirring sentence: *"The whole course of things goes to teach us faith."* I love this passage and remind myself of its profundity every day, especially when life sends me a curveball.

In an instant, I rejected the doctor's prognosis and resolved to prove him wrong. From that day forward, I decided to live only from a place of optimism. And although the next few months were ones of pain, I endured. Instead of wallowing, I attended lectures and read numerous books on the power of commitment in physical healing. I never let my faith waver in my ability to heal.

Six months later, when I visited my doctor for a follow-up appointment, he shook his head in bewilderment. "This just can't be," he said. "There is no sign of a fracture, and you seem to be in perfect health, free of pain. There must be some mistake. It's just miraculous."

Through my determination, along with the mind/body/spirit practices I'd learned from Fritzie, my back had managed to heal completely! Far from living a life of disability and chronic pain, I resumed fitness activities, and today I regularly participate in hiking, weight training, walking, biking, horseback riding, Pilates, yoga, and more.

I now see the accident as the impetus to changing my life for the better. My recovery proved that we have within ourselves everything we need to live life to the fullest. But we also need to learn from others who've walked the path we want to walk. I credit the individuals who shared their experiences through lectures, books, and conversations during that painful time as endowing me with the tools I needed to spearhead my own recovery.

Now, years later, I am at the other end of the spectrum, as my teaching, books, and life principles help others to live joyful, soul-satisfying lives. Gratefully, I now have an enthusiastic following and am in demand internationally as a health and fitness expert, personal growth specialist, leadership consultant, retreat leader, and motivational speaker for corporate, community, church, and women's groups. I strive to spread the message that ANYONE can choose radiant health and physical, mental, and spiritual rejuvenation. That's why I've written *Wired for High-Level Wellness*, so that you, too, can shape your own healing and live to your highest potential.

The sunflower has always been one of my favorite flowers along with tulips, roses, hydrangeas, and daffodils. I love how the sunflower's wide face is so open, how its yellow leaves brighten any room, and how, as a heliotrope, it naturally seeks the sun. I also love eating raw sunflower seeds and making sunflower seed milk and cheese (nondairy), and enjoy any salad, smoothie, or other dish that includes sunflower green sprouts as well. When I was a child I used to make up songs about sunflowers as they seemed like a natural companion to my own optimistic nature.

I was reminded of this connection recently when I heard a remarkable comment from a scientist being interviewed on the radio. He said, "Humans share 35% of their DNA with daffodils." I remembered again how much I felt the sunflower was almost an alter ego to myself and how fundamental our connection is to the natural world. Just as the sunflower turns its face toward the sun to grow and to thrive, so we each need to face the outer and inner light, always looking to the light of God, while also tending to our own budding seeds. We each blossom when planted in fertile soil and are fed nourishing food and care. We can be the caretakers of our own growth, just as we tend to our flowers, plants, pets, and other loved ones. Now is the time to let your newly nurtured roots gather strength in order to bloom.

Just like everything in nature, the body is in a continuous state of regeneration. It is constantly building itself up, tearing itself down, and rebuilding itself all over again. Exercising daily builds up strong muscles and bones; getting ample sleep builds up energy and vitality; eating a wholesome diet builds up immunity and revitalization; appreciating nature's beauty each day builds up a positive attitude; nourishing the mind with affirmative and constructive reading builds up the brain; and meditating/praying and reading the Bible daily builds up our spirituality and our connection to God.

How to Use This Book

As a holistic lifestyle coach for decades, I work with only a few select clients each year so that I can offer my utmost energy and vitality to each. Previous clients have included corporate presidents, politicians, world-class athletes, celebrities, and everyday people who want to achieve a greater sense of purpose. Working on all levels—physical, mental, emotional, and spiritual—I teach my clients how to incorporate my gold-star secrets to being vibrantly healthy and stunningly successful.

With a copy of *Wired for High-Level Wellness* in hand, think of yourself as one of my personal clients: You now have in your fingertips all my tools and advice to take your life from ordinary to extraordinary! Just for you, I have put decades of invaluable information and research into this reader-friendly book. I imagine you sitting across my kitchen table right now as we begin a friendly chat, one in which I wish to convey how much I want the best health possible for you, as well as inner peace. I hope you will understand how dearly I value these principles for myself and want to extend their benefits to everyone I know and care about—and that includes you!

Looking over the table of contents, you will see that the book is divided into six parts. Things worth doing are worth doing right, and so this is what I encourage you to do. Read through the book once quickly and then start back over and read more deliberately, reflecting on what you read and incorporating some of my tips and guidelines into your life as you see fit. In Chapter 15: Being Committed to Creating an Extraordinary Life, I am suggesting that you write out your new commitments (there's even a page in the book to do this) so you see them in front of you. Put simply, you want to . . . *Plan the work and work the plan.* From this book, you will find countless suggestions on how to enrich all areas of your life and they will only benefit you if you incorporate and practice them in your lifestyle and day-to-day routine.

If you want to be healthy, you can't treat your important desires and goals as afterthoughts. And I know it takes courage to make new changes in your lifestyle after years, and maybe decades, of living a certain way. We often resist change and gravitate to the familiar, even when we know it's not for our highest good.

You don't need to change *everything* at once. Baby steps, when consistent and enthusiastically embraced, will soon become your new normal. Feeling and looking better with all my simple, recommended changes is the greatest motivator. Remember, you need to have the courage not to squander a good thing—and, in this case, all the good things you will be reading about in this book. I know you have the courage and can achieve your goals. I believe in you!

Our Daily Choices

Our countless daily choices determine our level of health and how we feel. And there are three choices over which we always have control: what we eat, how we move (exercise), and what we think, and we have the power to change these at any time. And we also have the power to cultivate our dreams, and to celebrate each day. The power of choice is what living fully and successfully is all about.

The saying, "The ancients have stolen all our best ideas," remains true. What I'm writing about isn't really new; it's fresh only in that it's written from my perspective (combined with the wisdom of my grandmother and my mother) and daily experiences. For example, I pray and meditate every day, but on a few special days during the week, I couple this ritual with a sunrise hike. I am able to do this year-round because I have the privilege of living in sunny West Los Angeles, my native hometown. This is my time, when I let nature lift my spirit and nurture my soul. I always feel so close to God, Jesus, and my angels when I am outdoors reveling in Mother Nature's environment. As you'll see in this book, my sunrise hikes allow me to practice the principles of *exercising, being out in nature, appreciating beauty,* and *keeping my body hydrated and detoxified.*

I also regularly practice the principle of *not always taking myself and my life so seriously.* I simply love to laugh (I'm known to be a practical joker as David mentioned in his foreword)! My mother, June, called laughter "the body's elixir" or natural rejuvenator. It is an essential ingredient to daily living and something I use to fuel my spirituality. Because of my positive, easygoing, "lighten up" approach to life, I have acquired the nickname "Sunny" because I am always reminding others to not take life so seriously.

Boosting our self-esteem is a central theme throughout this book. No matter where I travel and with whom I work, on a universal level, I believe the thing people wrestle with most in their own lives is loss of faith in themselves—in other words, low self-esteem. In my own life, I fortify self-esteem through the principles of *filling my life with vim and verve, living a God-centered life, never letting anyone or anything cause me to doubt my ability to achieve my goals, staying committed to a healthy lifestyle,* and always *remembering that my body is God's temple and deserves to be treated lovingly—with respect and kindness.*

If we put God first in our lives and live with faith, greeting each day as a blessing, and treat ourselves with tenderness, our self-esteem will blossom. This is one of my favorite quotes about faith:

> **Faith is an invisible and invincible magnet, and attracts to itself whatever it fervently desires and persistently expects.**
>
> ~RALPH WALDO TRINE

These are just a few of the many suggestions I rely upon in my own experience and in my practice as a holistic lifestyle coach, teacher, and educator, and they are all my gifts to you in *Wired for High-Level Wellness.* You may not agree with my chosen path or what I write; all I ask is that you keep your heart tender and your mind open.

Books are more than just words on a page. You, the reader, bring the words to life. Apply what you read and look for ways you can experience more celebration and vitality in your life than you've ever felt before. I love what Henry David Thoreau said about the books he preferred to read:

> *Books, not which afford us a cowering enjoyment,*
> *but in which each thought is of unusual daring; such*
> *as an idle person cannot read, and a timid one would*
> *not be entertained by, which even make us dangerous*
> *to existing institutions—such I call good books.*

My hope is that this book cultivates this sense of "unusual daring" to take charge of your life in a powerful way. If you feel stuck or like you're in a "spin-cycle" lifestyle, if you've lost some of your joy and would like to experience more lasting happiness, or if you just need some gentle, loving, efficacious guidance to live in a more meaningful way . . . you will find the catalyst you need.

There is no time like the present. Make your life the magnificent adventure it was created to be. I salute your great adventure, and I wish you the daily feeling that you are *Wired for High-Level Wellness.*

The world is full of people who have dreams of playing at Carnegie Hall, of running a marathon, and of owning their own business. The difference between the people who make it across the finish line and everyone else is one simple thing: an action plan.

~JOHN TESH

It's daring to be curious about the unknown, to dream big dreams, to live outside prescribed boxes, to take risks, and above all, daring to investigate the way we live until we discover the deepest treasured purpose of why we are here.

~LUCI SWINDOLL

Part 1

Dream BIG
& Follow Your Heart

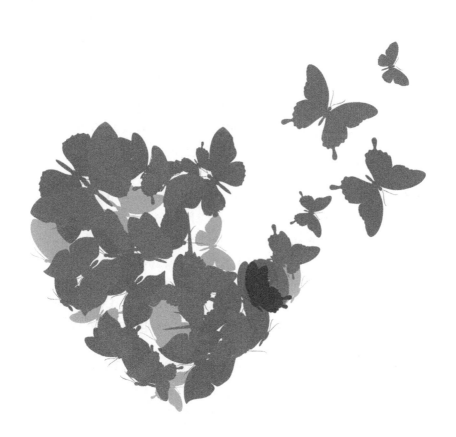

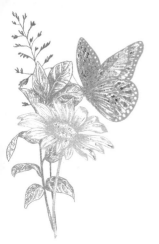

Chapter 1

Living with Purpose
& Celebrating Life
Along the Way

A truly good book teaches me better than to read it.
I must soon lay it down, and commence living on its hint.
What I begin by reading, I must finish by acting.

~HENRY DAVID THOREAU

As for God, His way is perfect; the word of the Lord is
tried: He is a buckler to all them that trust in Him.

~2 SAMUEL 22:31

As I travel the world giving talks and doing all kinds of media interviews (radio and TV talk shows, newspapers, and magazines), there are a few questions that seem to come up all the time for me to answer. One of them goes something like this: "Susan, you are such a prolific writer and your books are in multiple languages worldwide. How did you first get interested in writing and what were some of your life-changing experiences that guided you along the way in your chosen career path?"

So in this first chapter of the book, I will share with you how God kept my path brightly lit, starting from a very early age, and always encouraged me to walk in the direction of my dreams. So here we go on my personal journey . . .

Books have always been my friends. Like a single rose that can be my friend and a garden all by itself with fragrance indescribable, a single book can be my companion and security blanket at any time. My mom, June, and my grandmother, Fritzie, instilled in me the love of books and reading at a very young age. In my childhood bedroom, I devoted a special corner to my own personal library with beautiful books in full color that occupied my days and nights and always kept me company. I put some of my favorite passages from books on beautiful paper, decorating these pages with lots of colors and pizzazz, and then taped them to the ceiling of my bedroom so when I went to sleep, I could look up at the enchanting words.

I never felt alone growing up because reading gave me such joy and comfort and an imagination with no limits. Reading all kinds of books always inspired, enthralled, captivated, motivated, and empowered me. I remember telling my mom more than once that we needed to transform our entire home in a suburb of Los Angeles (yes, I am an LA native) into a beautiful library that everyone could visit often and borrow books. In all of June's love and willingness to keep my dreams and imagination alive, she would often respond with something like this: "Isn't that a great idea, Susie? I like how your mind thinks. Whatever you dream, you can create. And until we can fulfill your dream, let's go to our local library and different bookstores and get you some more books for your own personal library in your bedroom." That response always made me smile for hours.

Variety Is the Spice of Life

Through reading all kinds of books from the classics, to nonfiction and fiction, to travel guides and poetry, I could triumphantly journey in my mind to any place in the world—far and wide—without the slightest bit of limitation or hesitation. Copious reading expanded my imagination, and I learned to visualize the books' characters and put myself into the role of the heroines. Often in parts of fiction books I would read, I'd think about ways I could write it better or change the plot to a more fantastical or exhilarating storyline that worked better for my mindset. This practice came in very handy for me during my countless hours of babysitting, as you'll see below, when I made up stories to recite to the children.

When my friends would be outdoors playing and running around, I was often in my bedroom reading, and when I would join them outside, I'd usually be carrying one or more books with me. Instead of my parents and grandparents reading to me as a young girl, I would almost always insist on reading the books to them. Sometimes during these readings, I would stop and explain to them what the words meant to me. I know my family enjoyed lots of chuckles with my penchant for reading and books. Over and over I read my favorites, often memorizing the beautiful words and sentences and reciting them to other people. Words, and pages with words that had meaning, resonated in my heart as a young girl, and still do to this day. The fact that letters made into words, and words made into sentences, and sentences made into paragraphs that can create all kinds of emotions and deeply touch the heart, and literally help to transform lives and make the world a better place to live, is astonishing and so powerful to me. Through reading, we can feel happy, sad, positive, hopeful, joyous, upset, blissful, anxious, energized, invigorated, stimulated, vitalized, elated, and so much more.

If I were president of the United States, as you'd probably guess, I would make sure every school in America and every community had a commodious library, and I would find ways to give free books away to all children and to make it mandatory in all schools at all levels to incorporate in periods of reading time during the day and week.

Even at that young age, I developed a system of letting my friends borrow my books, one at a time, and they had to sign an agreement to return it in perfect condition within one week. I never lost any book and all my friends got on the bandwagon of book reading, too.

When my friends were sick and couldn't play, or their younger siblings were unwell, I would often call them up and read them books over the telephone to help cheer them up or make up stories to tell them. Ever losing interest in reading was an impossibility for me in my life.

Reading to Others

At my elementary school when I was in fifth and sixth grades, I was selected as the one person in the entire school who would visit the classrooms of the lower grades and read books to them. With enthusiasm and alacrity, I always relished these times of sharing my love of books and reading with other students. Not surprisingly, my friends gave me the nickname of "the book girl" since I was rarely without a book in my hand to read. And until the age of 14 when my aspirations changed, if anyone asked me what I wanted to do when I grew up, my most frequent answer was . . . "I want to be the best librarian in the world."

When I was a preteen and teenager, my mom would frequently volunteer at the local hospital. Of her many jobs, one was rolling around the book cart to each room to pass out books for patients to read. Early on, when I joined her, together we'd roll in the cart containing all kinds of books and it was the highlight of my day. After a while, I started giving a synopsis of the different books to help the patients select the best one for them, and those that had tired or weak eyes, I would gladly read to them. Before too long, I took over the book cart by myself, without my mom's help, and it was a joy indescribable to see the patients' faces beaming with delight when I read to them.

Even as a teenager, I was reading all of Jane Austen's magnificent books and loved each of them, especially *Pride and Prejudice*, first published in 1813. After multiple readings through the decades, the protagonist in that book, Elizabeth Bennet, still to this day, remains my favorite person in literature. With each of Austen's books, I would put myself into the role of the main female character and lived out the scenes in my mind and imagined that I was that strong, courageous, charming, and admired protagonist. What an absolute delight it was for me.

As an adolescent, I worked frequently as a babysitter with children of all ages, from the very young to early teens. Part and parcel of my babysitting accessories was my basket of books that I always carried with me so I could read to the children. If any one of them ever said to me that they wanted a new book or different and new story time, and I didn't have any extra books with me, I would make up all kinds of stories to tell the children. Each time I would lavishly regale the kids with imaginative, and always positive, stories about young people who were making their dreams come true. Sometimes my stories were about becoming a doctor, or scientist or renowned athlete. Other times my narratives were about being a ballerina or dancer, or an actor, or a princess or prince, or a veterinarian or even a chef, since I loved to cook with my mom and grandmother. Needless to say, I was the most popular and prosperous babysitter in my neighborhood and loved being around children of all ages, as I still do to this day.

Kids these days don't read like we did decades ago. That's an unfortunate fact, as I can't imagine not having books and reading when I was young. How grateful I still am to this day that my mom and grandmother engendered in me the love of reading. Most children I know these days are more into technology—computers, smartphones, and video games—than enjoying a book and turning the pages with glee as I always did. James Patterson said this and I agree with him: "The fact is that our kids aren't reading books—or frankly, much of anything lately. Schools are underfunded, some schools even closing their libraries. Parents have to realize that it's their job, and not the school's job, to get kids into the habit of reading for fun."

The Bible Is My All-Time Favorite Book

As I've gotten older, my love of reading has stayed with me for decades—which seem to have passed in the blink of an eye. I am still a voracious reader, amassing quite an impressive library in my home; I usually have around four to six books I'm reading at any given time all displayed on the table next to my bed. And I still read all kinds and genres of books. If I were asked which book I read the most, it would be the Bible, for sure. Several different editions beautifully occupy and shine brightly on an entire shelf of my library and my favorite Bible, given to me when I was a teenager by Fritzie, is always next to my bed.

Being outdoors in nature is one of my favorite activities, especially hiking in my local Santa Monica Mountains and other locations around the world, and also riding horses in wide open natural spaces and environments in the countryside, mountains, or along the beach. It's not uncommon for me to bring along a small book when I am hiking, riding, or simply sitting at the beach listening to the waves. To have a book while I'm basking in nature and experiencing the glory of perusing a book—an unbeatable combination to me—is sheer bliss.

And since I'm never without a book, I frequently read when I am in line at the grocery store, bank, DMV, post office, filling my car of gasoline or often at a restaurant when I am eating alone at a table. Having a book with me makes my solo dining experience most enjoyable. Many people get so frustrated and anxious when they need to wait in line. I enjoy waiting because it gives me another opportunity to fill my mind with inspiration that I derive from a book. In fact, there have been countless times when I would suggest that people behind me in line move in front of me so I can keep reading an enthralling section of the book or a page of poetry and see it through before I close the book up and put it away.

So, as you can see, it may not be so surprising to you that I now write books—over 33 of them to date (with more percolating in my mind) and many are printed in foreign languages. While I might not be able to read my books in different languages, it's still a tremendous sense of joy and accomplishment to see my writings perused around the world. Additionally, I have written thousands of magazine articles that have been read by millions of people worldwide.

My Writing Opened Doors of Adventure

As long as I can remember, besides reading books, I have enjoyed writing as well. Through writing, I have come to understand my life with more clarity and to appreciate the lessons that have been sent my way. Over the years, my life and my experience of being in this world have changed, just as I'm sure yours have. Expressing my thoughts and feelings on paper has frequently given me clues to how I might take care of unfinished business or unresolved conflict, and how I might identify the nugatory and troubling beliefs that keep me from being all I was created to be.

Writing articles and books has also brought me memorable consultations, speaking invitations, and more around the world with celebrities, businesspeople, and regular folks and families like you and me who are seeking to create a healthier, happier, and more balanced life. In fact, that's exactly how I met David Craddock. As he mentioned in his foreword, I was invited to give a few motivational, holistic health presentations in London, England, at a conference because the event coordinator read one of my articles in a magazine on simple ways to create a life of high-level wellness and he said it really inspired him. He reached out to me and extended an invitation to be one of the five conference speakers over the four-day event. How blessed I was that David also attended the conference, and you can read the rest of the story on how this serendipitous meeting with David changed our lives for the better in the previous forewords he has written in my books *Be the Change, Choose to Thrive, Invest in Yourself with Exercise,* and *Kitchen Gardening.*

One of the most memorable events in my life from someone reading my articles and books resulted in an invitation to speak about high-level wellness at a symposium in Aspen, Colorado, hosted by none other than John Denver. What I found out is that he had been reading and enjoying my magazine articles and books for years and extended an invitation to me to give two presentations at his first "Choices for the Future Symposium" in the mid-eighties. I had always been a huge fan of his music, so I was chuffed when I got the invitation. Over one thousand people from around the world attended this four-day event. Before the symposium started, all the speakers were invited to John's home for an afternoon and evening of conversation and gaiety.

I arrived at John's home and he greeted me kindly like we were old friends (it felt like we were), told me how much he enjoyed my writings, and encouraged me to keep writing more and more. He gave me a tour of his home and then, a cappella, sang me a song he had just written that no one in the public had ever heard titled "Falling Leaves." John also asked for some personal guidance on his diet and exercise program, which I gladly proffered. It was a wonderful time for me, and it all happened because he enjoyed my writings and wanted to meet me and welcome me as a speaker at his event.

Needless to say, my writings, whether in the form of books or magazine articles, have created a rewarding career and enriching life for me far surpassing my wildest expectations. Writing fills me with ineffable joy (even though it can sometimes be painful when the words are not flowing easily from my mind, heart, and soul), and I know I was born to be a writer, motivational speaker, and lover of nature.

Usually when I write, if I am not listening to the sounds of nature, I will have music on in the background that uplifts and inspires me and, yes, still to this day, it's often the music of John Denver along with others. If you are young and don't know who he is, I encourage you to check out his music. He was a wonderful songwriter and musician.

I'm Proud to Be a Logophile

There's something else I think you should know about me that will probably not surprise you after what I've just shared with you. I've always had a partiality for words, so much so that I have a dictionary in every room of my home. If I were stranded on a tropical island and could only take one additional book besides the Bible, without a doubt, it would be my dictionary. In fact, whenever I read a book—and I strive to read two to three books weekly—it only makes it to my list of favorites if it teaches me at least twelve new words.

Throughout the reading process, I keep a dictionary nearby to consult, and I often write the meaning of a new word, complete with its usage, derivation, and so on, right in the margin of the book. That way, if I'm ever rereading the book and forget the meaning of the word, the definition is right there on the page.

As you'll discover as you read my books, I've found special places to use some of my favorite, choice, yet often underused words. I hope you're willing to be stretched a little, too. Maybe you too will find yourself reading with a dictionary by your side and develop a fondness for looking up words that are new to you and becoming a wordsmith.

In all my books, I also aspire to communicate the love I have for life. In each one, I hope to share on a very personal level the lessons that have been most important to me. I see this as a voyage we'll take together, an adventure of hope, renewal, rejoicing and making choices. Your active participation is important, because it's not what we read that makes the difference in our lives but rather how we apply the ideas to ourselves. I love what Winston Churchill said about books:

If you cannot read all your books . . . fondle them—
peer into them, let them fall open where they will,
read from the first sentence that arrests the eye,
set them back on the shelves with your own hands,
arrange them on your own plan so that you at least
know where they are. Let them be your friends;
let them, at any rate, be your acquaintances.

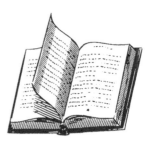

Designing a Library to Uplift & Inspire

I wanted to share with you one last story that may stimulate you to organize your home life and surroundings and upgrade your level of health. It was around 20 years ago and one of my clients, Bob, who lived in Brentwood (Los Angeles), had a magnificent collection of books and a huge home. Before I came into his life, he was totally out of shape—about 100 pounds overweight. He didn't know how to create healthy meals and usually ate takeout foods morning, noon, and night. He had never exercised more than stepping on the gas pedal in one of his many automobiles and had a grand home and gardens that were in total disarray. A few years prior, his parents and two sisters and only brother all passed away in the same year, and he spiraled into a deep depression and could hardly get out of bed most days. One of his closest friends suggested to Bob to call me up for a consultation to see what I could do to help lift him up and rejuvenate his home, body, life, heart, and soul again. So I arrived at his home the first week of January, walked through each room with him, and assessed the situation of how I could best support Bob to achieve his goals of getting fit, organized, happy, and hopeful again instead of being depressed and hopeless day in, day out.

In our first meeting after my home tour, we talked for about three hours about what he wanted to achieve and his time schedule to get everything done. His wish was that in one year, by Christmastime, he hoped to get to his goal weight with strength and muscle definition, have a home worthy of entertaining in and having friends over, and he also wanted a home gym and a special place for his collection of books. We met every day those first three weeks to go over my plans and to get things started and built. Fortunately, money was no object for Bob; however, he needed someone to deeply care about him and to take his goals and wishes to heart and bring his dreams to fruition. I told Bob that if he made the commitment and followed through on my training program, healthy new diet and nutrition program, and worked closely with me on his home reorganization and refurbishment, he would be living his highest dreams for himself within one year. I even asked Bob to sign a commitment contract with me that he would keep his word on everything he said he would do and always follow through. I'm a stickler for people keeping their word and doing what they say they will do without making up all kinds of excuses.

Plan the Work & Work the Plan

Since Bob had a huge backyard with extra space to spare, we immediately started building on an addition of a large home gym and also a library to house his thousands of books. We brought in an architect, a contractor, and construction crew with whom I had worked before who I knew always kept their words and always got jobs done on time or ahead of schedule—very rare in the world of construction.

While these additions were being built and ready to go, we started on his new exercise program, which included weight training, aerobics, Pilates, and other flexibility work. I also showed him how to do aerobic and strengthening exercises in his swimming pool as well as lap work, and taught him how to do floor work, which included planks, push-ups, crunches, and stretching.

For the first three months, I taught him all aspects of cooking and preparing healthy foods. (On page 240, you will find some easy, nutritious, and delicious recipes.) He purchased his first juicer and blender, and an Ionizer Plus Alkaline Water device for his kitchen and a Transcend Infrared Sauna—both from High Tech Health in Boulder, Colorado, and described in detail in my books *Choose to Thrive* and *The Curative Kitchen & Lifestyle* and also in detail on my website SusanSmithJones.com—where you can find out where to get these salubrious healthy living products that I wouldn't be without.

Since one of my many hobbies is gardening and doing landscape garden design, I created for him beautiful gardens for his front and back yards with water features. As the new home gym and library were both being built in Phase 1 "Setting Up a Salubrious Home Environment Program," I also tackled each room to refurbish and redecorate so he could have a home he was proud of and to warmly welcome guests that could stay over for a few days.

At the end of one month, he had already lost 22 pounds and was able to create a delicious meal for a few of his friends and me all by himself. Bob also requested getting a new wardrobe of clothes that fit him better. I recommended that we purchase only the bare essential clothing since he would still be losing another 80 pounds or so before the end of the year and would need better-fitting clothes for the entire year we worked together.

Yes, he achieved all of his goals in that year, and then some, and was feeling fully alive and thriving again. But here is another part to the story that's germane to the theme of this chapter and was so thrilling and breathtaking for me. Like me, Bob was also a collector of books but many of his books were rare treasures—first edition and autographed books that were worth a fortune and many of them were a couple hundred years old and more. One of his goals in life was to have an impressive home library and he asked me if I could bring his vision into manifestation. I told him of my love for books, too, and that his collection was the most magnificent reservoir of books I had ever seen. So I designed a spectacular library for him (the one that's been in my mind for years to build in my dream home one day) with the help of our architect and contractor that was made out of beautiful mahogany wood (that's a hard reddish-brown timber from a tropical tree that's used for high-quality furniture) and large enough to be a splendid home to his world-class book collection.

This project of the library was part of his Phase 2 "Rejuvenate Body

& Life Program," and after it was completed in five weeks, it then took me about eight months to totally organize the library in different categories and themes with many beveled-glass cabinets to house some of the oldest editions and, of course, a huge, hidden wall safe to provide cozy and luxurious accommodations for his most valuable, priceless books that only very special people ever got to see. Can you imagine how exhilarated I was to have this opportunity to look at each of these thousands of books, smell the pages, gently turn the old pages of his antique books (always wearing gloves, of course), and read words written long ago? It was one of my most amazing dreams come true to revel in Bob's sensational accumulation of books and organize them all to my liking in a library that would be easy for him and his guests to navigate. In this library, I also designed and had built a beautiful custom desk where he could work and read, and also a comfy couch and a couple reclining chairs. The final six weeks before I finished the library with all of the organization complete, Bob was out of the country so he didn't get to see the grand finale until he returned. When we walked into his completed library and he saw the end result, he actually cried with happiness because his new library surpassed his highest vision for himself. I certainly got a hero's welcome that day!

But that's not quite the end of the story. The following year, Bob built another home on the east coast in Florida that included a gym and another library about half the size of his library in Brentwood. He wanted to bring the overload of his books to be housed in his Florida home. Many of them could be shipped, but, understandably, he was not willing to ship some of his most valuable books and chance that they could be lost or stolen, so he was going to drive from Los Angeles to Florida with many of his most valuable books. When his Florida home construction was finished, Bob asked if I would come and see the home in person, finalize all of the interior design work, which, of course, included organizing his home's library and kitchen, and orchestrating his healthy living products and daily salutary practices. I could never pass up an opportunity to create another stunning library for him, this time made out of white oak, at my request.

A Road Trip Unlike Any Other

Of course, Bob was willing to fly me first-class to Florida after he arrived, but his first preference was for me to join him on the entire cross-country drive and keep him fit with daily exercise and help him with making healthy food choices during the trip. When he could tell that I wasn't so keen on taking the long drive with him, he sweetened the pot with doubling my daily salary and offering to put me in a beautiful suite in 5-star hotels each night with luxury spas, and this included any spa treatments of my choice at the end of each day's long traveling. Now he had my total attention, for sure! That plan sounded quite doable for me. Bob also arranged for us to see the Grand Canyon and many other natural sights. It was actually a wonderful way to see many parts of America up close that I had never visited before. We trained every morning, enjoyed healthy foods along the way, met countless lovely people, had spa treatments at night, and arrived in Florida healthier and more refreshed than when we left.

But here's one of the highlights of that cross-country trip for me and it had to do with words. A few of my goals on this trip were to keep my mind strong, to return home at the end smarter than when I left, and to make positive use of our time in the car with a few thousand miles of traveling. Bob had to agree to this idea I had for me to consent to share this trip-time with him and, happily for me, he wholeheartedly agreed for the reason that he was also a wordsmith. Since I was aware of the upcoming trip four months in advance of the departure date, I created about 600 cards (3 x 5) to learn new words and to better use words in general. On one side of the card, I put a word and its different derivations, and on the other side of the card, I put the definition and an example of using it in a sentence. Okay, I know what you're thinking—who in their right mind would travel across America and study vocabulary? It just happens to bring me great joy, and, fortunately, Bob also enjoyed this, too. We had a fierce competition going to see which one of us excelled the most in our word games.

For example, I created 100 cards (words) that every word lover should know and ways to use the words' different derivations in sentences (like *sesquipedalian*). I created another 100 cards that almost everyone confuses and misuses (like *lie* and *lay*). I created another 200 cards with each one highlighting words that make a difference and, on the opposite side, how to use them in a masterly way (like *peripatetic*). The next group of 100 cards I devoted to rare words and ways to master their meanings (like *pridian*). And in the final group of 100 cards, I featured words that are usually used in an incorrect way (like *displace* and *misplace*). None of this was onerous preparation work for me because I thoroughly enjoyed creating each card, which, as you probably already guessed, gave me a leg up on our vocabulary competitions while driving.

It goes without saying that both Bob and I had a better grasp of the English language and how to use words more accurately and masterly when our 3,200-mile trip from Los Angeles to the east coast of Florida was over. The only downside to this competition was that during the nights, I would often dream about words and could hardly turn off my brain from constantly analyzing all of my sentences and word usages when talking. Fortunately, Bob took great pleasure in our vocabulary contests and appreciated all of the long hours of work it took to get these vocabulary cards ready for our trip.

In addition to our vocabulary competitions, Bob also read to me from many of his rare, old books during the times I was driving. It was blissful to have these books and passages read to me. Reading in the car is not something I can do at length without feeling nauseous so Bob did all of the book and map reading.

By the end of our trip, each of use needed to come up with 33 of our favorite words—words that were a bit out of the mainstream and yet still have some utility in daily conversation or writing. Life is too short to use balderdash words. Here are the words from my list. I'll leave it up to you to look them up in your dictionary if you don't know their meaning.

1. Logophile*
2. Multifarious
3. Scintilla
4. Resplendent
5. Palaver
6. Erudite
7. Sagacious
8. Vituperative
9. Capricious

10.	Alacrity	18.	Perfidious	26.	Esoteric
11.	Antipathy	19.	Avant-garde	27.	Feckless
12.	Exigent	20.	Cacophony	28.	Scintillating
13.	Foment	21.	Elan	29.	Sequester
14.	Spurious	22.	Equanimity	30.	Ubiquitous
15.	Desultory	23.	Perspicacity	31.	Omniscient
16.	Fugacious	24.	Halcyon	32.	Nugatory
17.	Perspicuous	25.	Philistine	33.	Quintessential

*the perfect word for yours truly

God's Purpose for Our Lives

So as you can see, I was probably born to be a lover of words, reading, and writing. I am wired to write and to appreciate good books and beautiful words. It's who I am deep at my core. These passions of mine have helped to make my life a magnificent, splendiferous adventure.

My greatest hope is that reading this book will help you turn your life into a magnificent adventure, too. You do make a difference. There is no one like you in this entire world, no one with your talents, your eyes, your heart, your fingerprints, or your dreams. You are inimitable and have been given the puissance and potential to make your life, and this world, any way you want it to be. It doesn't matter where you've been, what you've done in the past, how many mistakes you've made, or how old you are. Right now, right this moment, you can begin to make different choices. You can choose to be all that you were created to be—vibrantly healthy, happy, God-centered, balanced, successful, and peaceful. You can feel totally alive, filled with enthusiasm for life, the way you felt when you were a small child—the way I felt as a young girl when I read books. Aliveness! Fully alive and thriving! It's a choice and it's your divine right.

As we spend some time together through the pages of this book, you will discover some of the ways I have chosen to live healthfully and what I think living a life of faith, confidence, joy, vitality, balance, vitality, and God-centeredness is all about. You will find out that it's more than just feeling fine physically. It's a joy and radiance for living such that each day and each and every moment can be a celebration.

My mission in life is not merely to survive, but to thrive; and to do so with some passion, compassion, humor, and style. Each day I want to find people and things to celebrate, move in the direction of my dreams, appreciate resplendent nature all around me, and open myself more fully to God's Love and Light and this miracle called life.

~SUSAN SMITH JONES

Truly I tell you, if you have faith as small as a mustard seed, you can say to this mountain, 'Move from here to there,' and it will move. Nothing will be impossible for you.

~MATTHEW 17:20

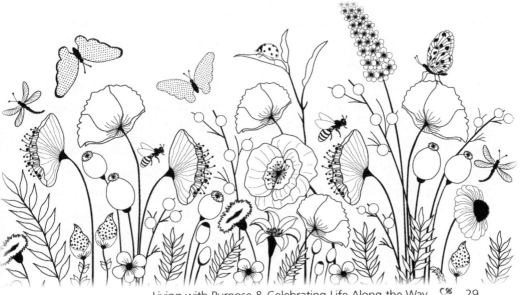

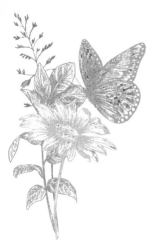

Chapter 2

Setting the Bar High

Whether you think you can,
or you think you can't—you're right.

~Henry Ford

Use hospitality to one another without grudging.

~1 Peter 4:9

*J*ust for a moment, close your eyes, breathe slowly and deeply a few times, and imagine yourself the master of the universe. As master you have the ability to create anything you want, even something that has never existed before. Be adventurous in your thinking, focusing on the result and not just the means, and envision what you most want now.

You have this power within you—it is the birthright and potential of every human being as a child of God. The only possible limitation is your own thought, belief, and imagination. Once you have a clear vision of what you want, then the natural play of universal forces will lead you to the accomplishment of that goal. Don't take your power lightly. Henry Ford knew all about it when he wrote, "Whether you think you can, or you think you can't—you're right." You, and only you, have the ability to create miracles in your mind and life. The choice is always with you. It has nothing to do with luck and everything to do with believing in yourself as a part of God's Divine Force that infuses and permeates everything in the universe. The great rule is this: if you can conceive it in your mind, then it can be brought into the physical world.

It takes boldness to go after your dreams, especially when you are exploring uncharted territory, but don't give up. When you compromise your dreams and values to live a life that is expected of you, rather than what your heart asks of you, you give away your power and disconnect from your soul.

"It takes a lot of courage to release the familiar and seemingly secure, to embrace the new," says my friend Alan Cohen, author of *Handle with Prayer*. "But there is no real security in what is no longer meaningful. There is more security in the adventurous and exciting, for in movement there is life, and in change there is power."

The world today certainly offers change, and it's easy to regard ability to keep up with the changes, perhaps even to cause changes here and there, as power. But power is drained, not created, by surviving in such a fast-paced world. The intense pace and stress of our daily lives can very easily put our peace, happiness, and health—not to mention our spiritual lives—at risk. When we're caught up in the whirl of today's hectic lifestyle, it's easy to forget the truth of our potential. We have less and less time for our own dreams, and in such circumstances our standards and values tend to deteriorate, leading to low self-esteem. It is when we feel that kind of inner emptiness that we are most tempted by any "quick fix" that comes along.

Life is hard, and learning to live with sacredness takes more time, but the fact is, we can slow things down. We can face our own challenges, however large or small, with aplomb and equanimity, on our own terms. We can choose to experience aliveness and become masters of our lives when we work closely with God. My hope is that this book will point the way to help you live your best life.

In the 1960s, psychologist Abraham Maslow wrote his famous *Toward a Psychology of Being*, which helped to change the entire emphasis of psychology. He chose to study high-functioning people—those living their highest potential—rather than people with problems, as was usually the case in psychology. Maslow developed a "psychology of being," which meant not striving but arriving, not trying to get someplace but living fully. Among all his high-functioning subjects, he found a common denominator. They all had a vision and were committed to it. They were self-motivated and believed they had the power to master life. That's one of the beliefs we will be working on throughout this book.

Do you believe you have the power to master life?

If It's to Be, It's Up to Me

Self-mastery begins with a complete and honest inventory of our lives. As Socrates so famously said, "The unexamined life is not worth living." Mastery involves taking responsibility for ourselves and what we've created, rather than blaming other people and circumstances for our lot in life. Blame is a convenient way of explaining why our life is not exactly what we would like it to be. The next time you start to blame another person or outside circumstances for how you feel or what you are experiencing, stop, check yourself, and remember: What you feel is up to you. Our feelings are governed by our mind. We can't think one thing and feel something else. Feelings and experiences always correspond to thoughts. If you are to become master of your life and live your highest potential, the habit of blaming others or circumstances has to stop. Setbacks and obstacles are only tests.

> *Do not be conformed to this world but be transformed*
> *by the renewal of your mind, that you may prove the*
> *will of God, what is good and acceptable and perfect.*
>
> ~ROMANS 12:2

Mastery involves being self-disciplined and courageous, moving through fear, recognizing our inherent Divine Power, and using it to bring our vision to life. Millions of masters-in-the-making, like you and me, are awakening to the concepts of self-responsibility and choice. The proof is in the success of teachers such as Joel and Victoria Osteen, Joyce Meyer, and others who help people bring spirituality and wholeness into everyday life. Once introduced to these empowering ideas, people give up being victims in favor of being masters. Self-mastery means becoming the heroes of our own lives.

Instead of whining, "Why?" and pointing the finger of blame, masters say, "This is the situation. I take responsibility for it. I realize I created this emotional stuff. I know I have the power to make new choices about how I view any event and how I react to it. I am powerful enough to 'uncreate' this situation and re-create something healthy and joyful. I now choose to see everything through the eyes of love. And with God as my ever-present source of love and support, anything and everything is possible."

Love empowers us. Nothing will transform and enrich life faster than the consistent experience of love. Let others know that you love them. Tell them and show them, often. Don't wait until later, for you don't know if they will still be here tomorrow. If we want to live our highest potential, all we have to do is teach the mind how to think differently—how to be gentle, thoughtful, relaxed, calm, loving, and centered on God. Seeing through the eyes of Love is the same as seeing through the eyes of God. Become comfortable with the idea that you are a spiritual being in a physical body, live from that awareness moment to moment, and your life will be transformed. It's simply an internal shift—a journey of mere inches from your mind to your heart. You will find yourself more certain, fulfilled, successful, content, and peaceful than ever before. You will be living in a state of grace.

Anyone who goes about living with a sense of serenity, contentment, and grace has no need to manipulate others. It is rare for a person who is reasonably satisfied with his or her own life to try to run someone else's. Such a person continues to grow through a living process of discovery and renewal and finds that self-mastery is the very opposite of control. As paradoxical as it may sound, this is the path to self-mastery: to surrender, trust, turn away from habits of accumulation, outer achievement, and quick fixes, and to allow one's sense of purpose to spring from inner guidance.

The more you live from inner guidance, the Christ Light—that peaceful, loving center within you—the more you'll find that everything you need to meet your wants and desires will be provided. The essence is in knowing that you are already whole and that nothing external to yourself in the physical world can make you any more complete.

Your Reality Reflects Your Thoughts and Intentions

We create our thoughts, our thoughts create our intentions, and our intentions create our reality. What you see around you, whom you associate with, how you function daily, what your relationships are like, how much money you make, how you get along with others, the shape of your physical body, and virtually everything about you is the result of your intention. Intention is directional energy, and intentional living is one of the most empowering ways to achieve happiness, health, and wholeness and to banish obstacles to spiritual growth. When life is lived with conscious intention, insights unfold more easily and everything proceeds more gracefully.

It is usually fairly easy to be happy and peaceful and to feel somewhat saintly when removed from social circumstances and relationships, but to be happy, peaceful, and balanced regardless of personal and environmental conditions is evidence of real spiritual growth. As you become more God-centered, your personal and environmental reality tends to adjust toward harmony. Your intentions reflect your values and spiritual beliefs back out into the world. If you view the world as a giving place, you probably see goodness in others and in all situations and are optimistic about other people's kindness and consideration. You usually find yourself surrounded by others with similar values. As a natural result, you experience much gratitude and are unconsciously teaching others to be more loving.

Our main job here on Earth is to take our focus and attention off criticizing and finding fault, and instead look for ways to serve others, share the peace and joy of our hearts, and let others know we appreciate them. When we continually find fault with someone, he or she withers up like a flower without water. Show love, respect, and appreciation to others and they will blossom. Isn't that what we all want—simply to be valued, appreciated, and loved?

Give this a try: for a day or two, treat others as if the fullness of

God resided within them. Imagine that their external attributes are nonexistent and that you can look directly into their hearts.

In any relationship with others, what really matters is the heart-to-heart or love connection. At the level of the heart, we are all connected by love, yet the love that connects us also makes us complete and whole beings within ourselves. The secret of relationships, whether they are with lovers, friends, or business associates, is to maintain our individuality in union. Remember that you are two selves. Let the winds of heaven dance between you always. Let Spirit guide you. The essence of who you are is Spirit. Spirit makes us all equally special and precious.

Being master of my life means that I put God first before everything. I choose to do this, trusting that my life's higher purpose is being revealed to me. My connection to God requires that I live my highest and best at all times and in all circumstances. I know the loving presence will give me the strength and courage to follow through on my commitments. Being centered on God also means that I give up depending on people, circumstances, and material things as my sources of happiness and fulfillment. I choose to put my faith in God and in my inner guidance.

Success Is an Inside Job

For years I have done research on what makes people successful. Along the way, I learned about Daniel Isenberg, who was a former professor at the Harvard Business School and a very popular teacher. He said that for years his former students would come back to him and say, "We really liked your courses, but now that we're out in the real world, what we learned at the business school doesn't seem to make much sense."

This bothered Isenberg because he wanted to teach his students something useful. So he obtained the names of the 25 most successful executives in the country and got permission to follow each of them around for a week to find out what it was they did that made them successful. Isenberg listened to their phone conversations, listened to them talk to their colleagues, friends, and families, and came to the conclusion that what made these people successful had nothing to do with what was taught at the business school. He discovered two important characteristics shared by all the successful people he observed.

One thing these achievers had in common was a commitment to putting their values first. There may come a time in our lives when our goals are in conflict with our values, a time when we want to do something in business or in some other connection, but we know it's a little judgmental or even a little unethical. We find ourselves torn between what we want to do at the moment and what we feel or know is right. What Isenberg's group of successful people had in common was loyalty to their values. They had learned that, without commitment to our values, either we don't achieve our goals, or if we do, they're not really worth achieving after all.

The second thing these highly successful executives had in common was an incredible faith in their intuition. They all exhibited spiritual sensibility. Some of them were churchgoers, some were not, but they all had a sense of a deeper intelligence in the universe that operated through them. Each of these people made decisions based on his intuitive feelings about what was going on in his or her business or professional life. We are all endowed with this "sixth sense" of intuition, but most people seem to rely on the other five senses, which usually interpret things according to their own likes and dislikes rather than according to what is true and beneficial for the soul. To know how to choose correctly in any given situation, we need to let the power of intuition guide our judgments.

How in tune are you with your intuition—with God's whisperings?

The Role of the Body in Self-Mastery

Living our best life means appreciating our magnificent bodies. The body is sacred, a temple of the living, loving spirit, and therefore deserves reverence. Treat yourself with respect. Don't wait until you're sick to recognize the miracle of your body. Honor the Light inside you and the Love you are. If you want to become healthier and more powerful, begin with how you feel about yourself, accepting your body as a temple. Heaven on Earth, our loving God, is inside each one of us at this moment. In your unique body, mind, and spirit you have been given everything you need to be the best you can be, to become master of your life. Cherish and respect your body unconditionally—no matter what its current shape—because it is sacred.

As children of God, Divine beings, we all deserve tender, loving care. We may find this difficult to accept, especially where our bodies are concerned. Many of us need to learn to be a friend to our bodies. Getting mad at our bodies only makes matters worse. Although they are but temporary homes for our spiritual being, we must still take care of them because they are sacred vessels for this voyage on Earth. Love your body and be committed to staying fit for your life journey.

Start today by tuning in more attentively to your body. It is a fantastic feedback machine. If you listen, you will discover that it communicates very well. When you get a headache, your body is trying to tell you something. Listen to your body's signals. The key is your willingness to listen and act. If you feel pain, what is your body trying to tell you? It may be telling you that you're eating too much, or eating the wrong kinds of food, or smoking or drinking too much, or not sleeping enough, or not drinking enough water or getting enough exercise. It could be telling you that there's too much emotional congestion in your life.

Listen to your body. Respect and appreciate it. Take loving care of it. You will learn to discern what your body is trying to tell you. And please, choose your doctor carefully. Choose someone who practices a wellness lifestyle and who listens to you. There is a tendency today for doctors to turn to technology and all kinds of elaborate testing, or to prescribe a regimen of medications, before listening to you or to their own intuition. I don't think it's a good trend. As you think about your health and health care, ask yourself these questions: "What can the doctor do for me?" and "How can I help myself?" You are the authority on your body. Educate yourself. If you have specific health conditions, read up on them online and figure out how to get the best possible care. And remember this: It is normal to be healthy. It's your divine birthright to be well.

Love Is the Main Ingredient to Living Your Best Life

One of the most powerful things you can do for your health is to love yourself unconditionally, every day. Treat yourself with respect and dignity. These are the simplest ways to experience peace and the joy of living. It may sound too simple, but I urge you to consider the power of self-love. Remind yourself constantly, so you won't forget. Stick notes on the refrigerator and the mirrors around your home if you need to that read, "I love myself" and "I treat myself with the utmost dignity." Erich Fromm said, "Our highest calling in life is precisely to take loving care of ourselves." When you change your attitude about yourself from negative to positive, everything else in your life will change for the better.

> When you change your attitude about yourself from negative to positive, everything else in your life will change for the better.

One of the extraordinary secrets of this world is that life flows outward. It originates inside and is projected outward, where it is perceived as the external world. People and situations and circumstances don't affect us unless we allow them to. We are affected only by what happens inside us, how we process situations, interactions, and events. We are affected only by our own feelings and our own thoughts. Nothing outside has the power to affect us.

Most people denigrate themselves all the time, in fun or in earnest. Beware, because in doing that, especially out loud or publicly, you create your own problems. If you think that somebody else hurts you or makes you happy or that some other person makes you feel good or bad about yourself, it's a delusion. Nobody else is responsible for your pain or pleasure. Nobody else is responsible for your sorrow or joy. You are the only one who can change what you think and how you feel. Make it a personal policy never to put yourself down. Never debase yourself or think negatively about yourself. Tune in to the inner guidance, the loving presence of Christ within you, that is with you 24/7 and realize that you are whole and wonderful and powerful beyond measure.

When you get in touch with your innermost Divineness and come in contact with that infinite, Christ-Light that is always a part of you and your daily life, you know what you should think, do, and say. Embrace your feelings—all of them. Pay attention to what your body, mind, and Spirit are telling you. You are getting messages all the time. For example, let's say you have made a commitment to only speak and think positive words and thoughts about yourself and your body. Then you find yourself walking by a store window and you see a reflection of your body in the window. The distortion of the glass expands your size. For a moment you cringe, and then your internal voice starts blathering out denigrations such as "I'll never be able to get down to my ideal weight" or "If only I had smaller hips and thighs" or "I wish I looked like the women on the TV show *The Real Housewives of* _____" or "That's it, I'm so depressed at how I look today that I think I'll wait until next Monday to start fresh and will just eat whatever I want for the rest of this week." When something like this happens, focus directly on what is right in front of you, your goal, and the truth of your being. Bring your thoughts back to the positive. Direct your attention to the things you appreciate about yourself and your body. For example, "Would you look at that! My legs are strong enough to carry me past this store window, and my eyes see God's child in my reflection." Or "I am walking with a bounce in my step and am delighted to have the energy to carry me forward in my daily activities." When any experience keeps repeating, this is a signal demanding further attention.

Don't be afraid of darkness, of dark or negative feelings, for darkness is the harbinger of light. "The dark night of the soul," says Joseph Campbell, "comes just before revelation. When everything is lost and all seems darkest, then comes the new life and all that is needed." In other words, sometimes things need to fall apart in our lives in order to come together again and unfold at a higher level. To make that happen, turn everything in your life over to the power of God within you, and surrender it all. That Christ-Light and Love within you exists within everybody but is being wasted by those who don't take the time to turn within. You may not find it easy at first, but everybody can do it with practice.

For example, even though you might have recently made a commitment to create more prosperity in your life, or meet new friends, or detox your entire body, it's not uncommon for the "appearances" in those specific areas to seem to get worse. In fact, when you're detoxifying, as you will read about in Chapter 5, your body goes through a house-cleansing and you might experience a few days of feeling worse before you feel better. If you choose to say hello to strangers on the street or at office or social gatherings, you might experience many cold shoulders before you find a tenderhearted person with whom you would like to create a friendship. I always look at everything as Spirit's way to keep me heading in the right direction.

> I trust that everything will unfold perfectly when I keep my intentions and goals directly in front of me and choose to live a God-centered life.

Divinity Is Another Main Ingredient

A most useful way to begin each day is with prayer and meditation (refer to Chapters 7 and 8 for more details on the history of meditation and how to do it).

I urge you to make meditation a top priority in your life. Don't mystify it. The process of meditation is nothing more than quietly going within and discovering your highest self—the presence of God within you. Meditation also allows you to empty yourself of the endless activity of your mind and to attain calmness. Regular meditation has many benefits. It is a natural way to attain peace of mind: it strengthens the body's immune system, slows the biologic aging process, awakens regenerative energies, enlivens the nervous system, and enhances creative abilities. Meditation will enable you to be more peaceful, soul-centered, and aware of the spiritual dimensions of your life. With progressive spiritual growth, you will be more insightful and more intellectually and intuitively capable of discerning the difference between truth and untruth. Ultimately, when you adopt meditation as a way of life, you'll be able to go to that peaceful place within yourself anytime and carry that peace and joy to all the circumstances in your life.

Listen to Franz Kafka: "You do not need to leave your room. Remain sitting at your table and listen. Do not even listen, simply wait. Do not even wait, be quiet, still, and solitary. The world will freely offer itself to you to be unmasked, it has no choice, it will roll in ecstasy at your feet."

Once you make a routine of daily spiritual practice, look for the proof of its value in how you live every waking moment. It is in the arena of everyday circumstances and relationships that we are provided with opportunities to explore the depth and clarity of our understanding.

How we experience life is a direct reflection of our inner condition, of our psychological health, maturity, understanding of our reason for living, and willingness to do what it takes to live successfully.

As important as it is to develop a spiritual practice, it is equally important not to become addicted to it or to indulge yourself in inner work to the exclusion of meaningful activities and relationships. Be sure to balance your regular sessions of meditation, inner reflection, and prayer time/Bible reading with worthwhile involvements in your outer life. In this way you fulfill yourself and your purpose in life.

> Meditation is a natural way to attain peace of mind. It strengthens the body's immune system, slows the biologic aging process, awakens regenerative energies, enlivens the nervous system, and enhances creative abilities.

If this all sounds high minded, remember this: It doesn't matter if you've never done it before. It doesn't matter what your level of health or spirituality is right now. At any moment you can choose differently. You can use your past mistakes or poor choices and learn from them. In fact, some people have to be at the very bottom before they awaken to the fact that they can choose something else. This is exactly what happened to a friend of mine, Mary June. I briefly covered this story in a previous book, but here is the whole story.

Mary June's Transformation

As the sun was shining over Santa Monica Bay, with its panoply of luscious colors illuminating the sky and the water, I was skating on the bike path, oblivious to people playing on the beach or passing by me. Alone and pensive, caught up in the fluid motion of my body and mind harmoniously in sync, I felt a palpable peacefulness—so often fleeting in today's stress-filled lives—infusing every cell in my body and permeating my thoughts. The melodious syncopation of the waves caressing the sand accompanied each stride.

And then it happened. What felt like a gigantic rock—it was actually only a quarter-sized stone—caught a wheel of my in-line skate and down I went, slamming into the cement. Fortunately, at that moment no one was there to see my less-than-graceful descent, except for a woman sitting on a bench about ten feet away. She immediately came over to make sure I was okay. Her gentle kindness and amiable countenance immediately comforted me. She helped me to the bench, where I removed my helmet. When I saw the jagged lacerations on the helmet, I felt overjoyed and grateful that I had worn protection and that nothing in my body was broken—just a few minor scratches and abrasions on my arms and legs and some major bruises to my ego.

As I got myself under control and determined that I could skate back to my car, I focused my attention on the sympathetic woman by my side and noticed from her swollen, bloodshot eyes that she had been crying. Feeling I could help, I invited her, after exchanging a few niceties, to have lunch with me, and she acquiesced. So I skated to my car and we met a few minutes later at a nearby restaurant.

We all have difficult and sometimes heartbreaking stories to tell, and Mary June (MJ) was no exception. Over a three-hour lunch I learned, in a nutshell, that MJ's two children had been killed by a drunk driver less than a year before. Soon thereafter she discovered that her husband was having an affair with his assistant, who was 25 years his junior. He had recently served her with divorce papers—just weeks after they had learned she had breast cancer. Then, a couple of days before we met, she had been let go from her job because of all the time she had been absent from work, owing to the necessity for medical care.

Through all the twists and turns of her recent life, MJ had kept a remarkably optimistic attitude and ability to rise above her challenges and had been able to hold onto a childlike trust and belief that there had to be some Divine order to it all. I learned that only minutes before my fall, sadness had overcome her and she had been crying, grieving the loss of her family and husband, her breast, her job, and everything about the normal life she thought was hers only a year before. It would have been easy to see herself as a victim and sink into despair, and most people she knew would not have blamed her, but MJ believed there was another, better way.

Fortunately, MJ had enough money to live for a few months without needing to work. Her only goal now was to create a healthy, balanced lifestyle and find ways to nurture her body, mind, and spirit. She told me that she wanted to lose weight and get back into shape, simplify the clutter in her house and beautify her surroundings, learn to meditate, plant a garden, and find some good books to read to nurture her new holistic lifestyle, but she didn't know where to start.

At that moment I discovered why my angels had made me fall practically at her feet. Until then, she was not aware of my work, books, and passion for motivating others to live their highest vision. When she found out about what I did and that I was giving a three-hour workshop that same evening called "Celebrate Life: Rejuvenate Body, Mind & Spirit with Empowering Disciplines," we both laughed until we cried. What a providential encounter it was, and what a powerful lesson for both of us that we're always in the right place at the right time and are constantly being guided and cared for by a loving Presence. Only minutes before I crashed into her world, she was asking God for the right direction to take and the best person to guide her in living a more healthy, balanced lifestyle.

Over the next three months, I was MJ's holistic lifestyle coach. We started by writing out her goals and dreams and creating affirmations to support her highest vision for herself. She immediately implemented a well-rounded exercise regime, which included aerobics, strength training, and flexibility exercises. In her home, we started with the kitchen and cleaned out anything and everything that wasn't for her highest good, nearly emptying the cupboards, pantry, and refrigerator. We went shopping at the local health food store and the supermarket so that she'd have healthy foods in her home from which to choose.

Next, we cleaned out every drawer and closet in her home (my passion for simplifying, organizing, and beautifying our surroundings has resulted in a fulfilling side business I call "Simply Organized"), added cheerful shelf paper here and there, and brightened some walls with new paint. We extended the theme of brightening and adding more color by creating two lovely gardens in the front and back of her home, where nothing but weeds had grown. As an amateur horticulturist and landscape designer, I relish getting my hands in the soil, planting a variety of greenery, flowers, and trees, and working with the nature angels to create a natural, celestial environment that will attract birds—especially hummingbirds—and butterflies. I even persuaded MJ to add a fountain to her yard and bring a couple more into her home as a way of fostering tranquility and serenity. Finally, I taught her how to meditate, a discipline that she took to like a butterfly to buddleia (a butterfly-loving plant!).

MJ made a conscious choice to surrender her life to God and commit herself to being the best she could be. Within six months, she was down to her ideal weight, having lost 33 pounds, and was fitter and healthier than she had ever been in her life. After taking a few classes in interior design, a dream of hers since she was young, she started working part-time as an assistant to a prominent designer in Santa Monica. Because of her courage and assiduity, her healthy diet, a positive and balanced lifestyle that nurtures her body, mind, and spirit, and a support team of doctors and friends, MJ feels confident that neither cancer nor any other degenerative disease will ever be part of her life again. And when she least expected it—as she was working out in the gym—she met a loving, upstanding man who shares many of her interests and has asked her to go with him on a long trip to Europe.

I have no doubt that our meeting was divinely guided for our mutual empowerment. I helped her transform and enhance her life; MJ profoundly inspired and motivated me with her integrity, willing spirit, and devotion to making her life better. She realized that "If it's to be, it's up to me" and took responsibility for her own happiness and fulfillment. She has discovered her purpose, followed her heart, and begun living with authentic power and passion. MJ and I both learned firsthand that breakthroughs and miracles occur when we're willing to live our vision and commitment.

The Power of Commitment

Lack of commitment is like an epidemic in our society. Just look around. People say they're committed to creating a healthier, more harmonious planet, yet they continue to litter, don't recycle, and drive cars that pollute. They say they're committed to their relationships, yet they lie, are unfaithful, are unwilling to be vulnerable, or walk out at the first sign of difficulty or challenge. They say they're committed to aligning with the spiritual side of their natures, but they set aside no time for meditation, solitude, Bible-reading, or communion with God.

Many people wish they felt more committed and wish they had something really big to commit to. They don't realize that the first big commitment has to be to themselves. By really committing to your best self and following through on your convictions and decisions, you will gain tremendous power. Nothing can keep you from becoming master of your life.

When you're committed to your health, you allow nothing to deter you from reaching your goal and are disciplined even when you're not feeling motivated. Discipline is the ability to carry out a resolution long after the mood and enthusiasm have left you. Of course there were times when MJ didn't feel like making a healthy dinner or getting up early to exercise after she had stayed up late to see a movie or visit friends, but she harnessed that inner commitment and persisted in keeping her word to herself. And on those few occasions when she experienced setbacks, instead of beating herself up with guilt and anger for doing something unhealthy, she came to see that these were choices from which she could learn and perhaps make better ones the next time. As she began to pay close attention, she noticed that splurging on unhealthy food made her feel lethargic for the next few days and she quickly came to realize that the momentary taste pleasure wasn't worth hours and days of feeling sluggish and morose. This is how we change: by paying attention and by our commitments.

When we make a commitment, we are willing to put all of our resources on the line and take responsibility for the outcome. Commitment—to a project, a relationship, or a health and fitness program—brings stability to the chaotic whirl of everyday life. Daily acts that reaffirm the commitment will increase our feelings of empowerment and self-esteem. The better MJ felt about herself, the more easily she made choices that were for her highest good, like going to the gym earlier than usual some mornings because of a busy schedule, or like choosing to eat more colorful, plant-based foods and drink more water and fresh juice even when she yearned to eat something unhealthy.

> Discipline is the ability to carry out a resolution long after the mood and enthusiasm have left you.

Through our everyday behavior we learn what really counts. Commitment, like peacefulness, must be woven through all of life, through our thoughts, emotions, words, and actions. I often hear people say they are committed to being healthy, yet they continually let things get in the way. They say they'll have to wait "until next Monday or the day after" to exercise because they're "just too busy now," even though they've made a commitment to exercise every day. Or they won't be able to start eating nutritious meals for the next two weeks because of birthdays, anniversaries, travels, or because they are "just too stressed out" to make a major change right now.

Commitment means that you get past your excuses and follow through on what you said you were going to do. Make your word count, especially your word to yourself. How can you ever expect someone else to make a commitment to you, and how can they ever expect you to follow through on a commitment to them, unless you show that you can keep a commitment to yourself? If you are committed, you arrange your personal circumstances so that your lifestyle supports your commitment. You can and will do whatever it takes to put your life in order, let go of excess baggage and nonessentials, and consciously focus on what is important.

Turn Adversity to Advantage

In my life and the lives of many people I know, the most growth, the greatest lessons, and the most rewarding transformations have always sprung from the greatest adversities and challenges. MJ's experience is a perfect example. If we haven't worked through or learned from these challenges, they have a way of reappearing in more damaging form. But once we've heeded the message and committed to changing our course, life has a way of making certain past misfortunes pay extra dividends. I'll bet you know exactly what I mean.

Here's an example from my life: A few years ago I signed a multi-book contract with a major book publisher. The second book in the series needed to be written more quickly than was comfortable for my balanced living lifestyle. It meant that I needed to curtail all socializing for over three months while I focused on writing the book and on my other work responsibilities. I explained the situation to my friends and told them that I would only be able to see them if they were willing to come with me on my early morning hikes. Well, very few (in fact only two) friends agreed to visit with me early mornings, but they did end up accompanying me regularly for sunrise hikes. These visits turned out to be the highlight of my week. We discussed issues I was addressing in the book, which in turn made it much easier to write when I sat down at my computer. During this same period I was invited to appear on a prestigious national television talk show. It would have required a few days of travel and work, and I didn't see how I could take that kind of time away from my writing. When I thanked the producer and asked her to check back with me in two months, she just laughed. She thought I was joking.

For days, I was filled with doubt, wondering if I had made a big mistake. But life, as I say, has a way of rewarding us for taking care of ourselves. Once the book was released, I sent it to the same producer. She called immediately and offered me an even greater TV opportunity.

She also told me that she applauded my commitment to my goal and how I let nothing stand in the way to bringing it to fruition. She said that my decision to forego her first TV offer gave her pause and ended up being a catalyst for her to be more focused in her work and personal commitments. In fact, those were some of the very topics that we discussed on the TV show when I finally arrived and participated.

Blaming, complaining, and taking no action only keeps us in a rut. It is important to always look beyond how a situation appears and to choose to see our lives from a higher perspective. The secret is to view everything around you as an aspect of yourself. In this way you shatter the illusion of separation and with it the need to blame and complain.

If you are feeling stuck, ask this question: "What is it I need to learn to finish this business so I can move on in my life?" Choose to turn adversity into opportunity by taking responsibility for everything you've created in your life and accepting the consequences of your choices, both good and bad. It gets you nowhere to transfer blame to other people or circumstances. You must be willing to accept whatever happens as the product of your own thoughts and actions.

Accepting responsibility can feel very burdensome and scary, I know. When I began taking responsibility for everything I was or wasn't creating in my life, I was scared. If my life wasn't working, I had no one to blame but myself, and that felt awful at first. But soon I realized that taking responsibility was also very empowering and freeing. I could steer this ship any way I wanted! This is what living is all about—mastering our lives by becoming all that we were created to be.

Try to avoid making routine matters and everyday relationships complicated. Your life is your gift to yourself and to the world through thoughtful service to others. Knowing this, I encourage you to unfailingly and enthusiastically welcome each day with joy and thankfulness because of the limitless opportunity it offers to learn, grow, flourish, and be truly happy and fulfilled, even—no, especially—if it feels hard to do. If this approach to each new day is not already a habit with you, make it your first priority from now on. Practice the presence of Spirit. Choose to look for God in every situation and circumstance in your day.

Look deep within yourself to get in touch with the truth of your being and the unlimited possibilities that await you. To assist in the process, you may want to ponder these questions and thoughts, as I had MJ do at the start of her commitment program.

PERSONAL COMMITMENT STATEMENT

Complete—on paper—the following statements:

❖ This is how my life would be if I were now living my highest vision:

❖ I commit to do the following to make my vision my reality:

❖ These are the ways I will now rearrange my lifestyle in order to support my commitments:

❖ The non-useful behaviors I will discontinue are:

❖ The new, constructive behaviors I will implement are:

❖ I will nurture my spiritual self by:

Write out the following Personal Commitment Statement or Positive Affirmation beneath your answers and read it out loud and with feeling. Sign your name, and date it. Reread it often. This is your positive personal commitment. From time to time, as you achieve your goals and live your vision at higher levels, you will want to rewrite and refine your Personal Commitment Statement or Positive Affirmation.

I am passionately, unshakably devoted to my vision of how I want my life to be. I am committed to making my vision a reality, for I know I have the power and ability to live my vision. Everything unlike my vision is dissipating, easily and effortlessly. I agree and affirm that I will do my best to help myself to total wellness and spiritual growth, and I will share my increasing radiance with my world. What I sincerely desire for myself I also see and allow for others. Thank you for this precious gift of life. Today, as always, I honor and serve God (Spirit) by loving myself and everyone else unconditionally and by acknowledging Spirit's presence in everything I think, feel, say, and do.

Make a Difference

You can make a profound difference in other people's lives by the way you choose to live yours. I'm reminded of the story of a young boy who was walking down the beach, picking up starfish, and throwing them out into the waves. A man watched him for a while and finally caught up with the youth. He asked, "What are you doing that for?" The boy answered that the stranded starfish would die if left in the morning sun. "But the beach goes on for miles and there are millions of starfish," countered the man. "How can your effort make any difference?" The boy looked at the starfish in his hand, threw it hard back into the sea, and replied, "It made a difference to that one!"

It makes a difference to those around you when you are loving, peaceful, happy, and healthy. It makes a difference every place you go when you are master of your life. You make a difference.

Our bodies are made up of billions of cells. To maintain optimum health, each of these cells must operate at peak performance. When we have sick or weak cells, the stronger, healthier ones must work harder so that our body as a whole will be healthy. Consider that the human race is like a body, and we are each its individual cells. If we are all cells in the same body, then ultimately we are not separate from others. There is no room for negative thinking, lack of forgiveness, hubris, bitterness toward others, or selfishness. It is our responsibility to this global body to be a healthy, happy, peaceful, loving cell that radiates only goodness, positivity, and joy. Think of it as contributing to the health and harmony of the whole world.

> It makes a difference to those around you when you are loving, peaceful, happy, and healthy.

For too long, our thoughts and beliefs regarding our life on this planet have been colored by artificial divisions. It is time we examined and corrected them. To create peace on Earth, we must stop dividing the world—the nations, the races, the religions, the sexes, the ages, the families, and the resources—and realize it is time to live together in peace, forgiveness, and love. Awareness that we are one must precede all our thoughts and actions as a part of our belief system. We are all connected to one another and to this living, breathing planet. We have a choice, and we can choose to make a difference with the way we live our lives.

In his book *The Hundredth Monkey*, Ken Keyes, Jr., tells of a phenomenon observed by scientists. The eating habits of macaque monkeys were studied on several islands. One monkey discovered that sweet potatoes tasted better when she washed them before eating them. That monkey taught her mother and friends until one day a certain number (ninety-nine, to be exact) of the monkeys knew how to wash their sweet potatoes. The next day, when the hundredth monkey learned how to wash sweet potatoes, an amazing thing happened: the rest of the colony miraculously knew how to wash their sweet potatoes, too! Not only that, but the monkeys on other islands started washing their sweet potatoes as well. Strange, but true.

> We're here on Earth not to see through one another, but to see one another through.

Keyes applied this "hundredth monkey" phenomenon to humanity. When more of us individually choose to make a difference with our lives—when human beings realize we each make a difference and start acting as though we do—more and more of us will learn this truth until we reach the "millionth person," and peace and cooperation will spread across the globe. I believe that, although we can't change the world, we can choose to know and change ourselves and that as we do, the world will be different. We will truly be masters of the universe—not by controlling one another, but by being masters of ourselves all together.

We're here on Earth not to see through one another, but to see one another through. We are here to experience the fullness of life. We are here to become the best we can be. We owe it to ourselves. As we change ourselves, we change the world. In one of his TV sermons, I heard Joel Osteen say, "Life's too short to spend it trying to keep others happy. You can't please everyone. To fulfill your destiny, stay true to your heart." He also said, "God would not have put a dream in your heart if He had not already given you everything you need to fulfill it."

*I know that there is nothing better for people than
to be happy and to do good while they live.*

~ECCLESIASTES 3:12

*If you can think of yourself as being all that you know you
should be: constant, gentle, loving and kind to every man,
woman, and child, and to every circumstance in life; kind and
tolerant in your attitude towards all conditions on earth;
Above all, if you can conceive yourself as being completely
calm in all conditions and circumstances, quiet and
yet strong—strong to aid your weaker brethren,
strong to speak the right word, to take the right action,
and so become a tower of strength and light;
If you can see yourself facing injustice and unkindness with
a serene spirit, knowing that all things work out in time for
good, and that justice is always eventually triumphant;
If you have patience to await the process of the outworking
of the will of God; if you can picture becoming like
this, you will know something of mastership.*

~WHITE EAGLE, THE QUIET MIND

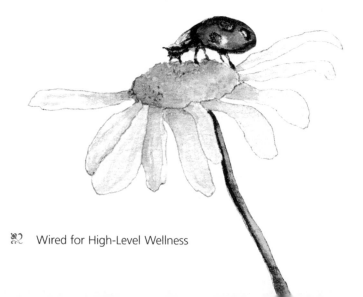

Part 2
High-Level Wellness
at Any Age

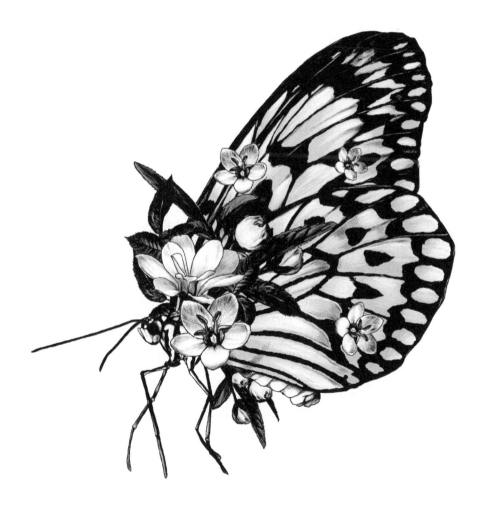

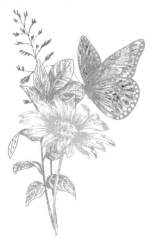

Chapter 3

Keeping Your Brain Sharp & Healthy

Be of good comfort, be of one mind, live in peace;
and the God of love and peace shall be with you.

~2 CORINTHIANS 13:11

This is my simple religion. There is no need for temples;
no need for complicated philosophy. Our own brain,
our own heart is our temple; the philosophy is kindness.

~DALAI LAMA

*P*eople often joke about getting older and forgetful, but it's not a laughing matter. A hit-or-miss memory and issues such as brain fog can really put you off your game, and as usual, oxidative stress is the culprit.

When we are young, our brain and mind are sharp and focused and our memory is keen. As we get older, however, we assume that we will start becoming forgetful, have a hard time finding the right words to express, and lose our personal belongings somewhere in our home. We presume that brain fog will be our "new normal" as we get up in years, and many of us have seen this happen with loved ones and friends. But it doesn't have to be that way. You can be as mentally clear and perceptive in your seventies and beyond as you were in your forties and fifties, and this chapter will cover some of my tips for brain vitality.

What Is Brain Fog?

Brain fog, also commonly known as brain fatigue, mental fog, and clouding of consciousness, can be a mild to severe episode of mental confusion that can strike without warning. When this occurs, it is common to experience a lack of focus, poor memory recall, and reduced mental acuity. If the underlying causes of the brain fog are not addressed, then the condition can continue to occur to the point that it can negatively affect one's professional and personal life.

Common Causes of Brain Fog

Brain fog and fatigue can be caused by a range of factors. In all cases, getting to the heart of what causes the brain fog is the key to overcoming this debilitating condition. Common causes of brain fatigue include:

❖ **TOXIC BODY**: Brain fog is one of the first indicators of a toxic body. Year-round, keep your body detoxified (on the alkaline side instead of being more acidic) by supporting the organs of elimination, including the skin, lungs, kidneys, and bowel. For thorough, effective, whole-body detoxification, the most valuable program is to combine the Transcend Infrared Sauna and Ionizer Plus Alkaline Water—both described in detail on my website SusanSmithJones.com

❖ **LACK OF SLEEP**: The brain needs sleep to recuperate. So when sleep is regularly interrupted, or when one suffers from a sleep disorder, he or she is more likely to experience brain fog in the morning upon waking. For some, a simple cup of coffee is enough to clear away the fog (freshly made alkaline water with lemon works for me by itself and in any recipe requiring water), but for those who suffer from serious sleep deprivation, the fog can stay for quite some time.

❖ **NEUROLOGICAL DISORDERS**: Certain neurological disorders have brain fog as side effects of the condition. These include fibromyalgia, lupus, chronic fatigue syndrome, and multiple sclerosis.

- ✤ **STRESS**: Stress is very powerful, and it can negatively affect the body in a number of ways, including causing brain fatigue. While this is common during times of severe stress, such as when a loved one passes or a relationship breaks up, normal everyday stress should not cause it. If one starts experiencing brain fog from normal everyday stress, this may be an underlying sign of another problem.

- ✤ **MENOPAUSE**: When women go through menopause, they sometimes experience brain fog due to fluctuating hormones. As the hormones become regulated, the symptoms of brain fog tend to disappear.

- ✤ **DIABETES**: Since glucose is the primary source of energy for the brain, fluctuating glucose levels in the blood can cause some short-term brain fatigue symptoms. For this reason, those with diabetes are at high risk for brain fog.

- ✤ **NUTRITIONAL DEFICIENCIES**: Strong brain function relies on proper levels of magnesium, vitamins B12 and D3, and amino acids in the body. When these nutrients are deficient or the body is dehydrated, brain fog can occur.

- ✤ **SIDE EFFECTS OF MEDICATIONS**: Certain medications, such as those for high blood pressure, pain management, and allergy relief, can cause mental confusion as a side effect. This can occur with any type of medication, both prescribed and over-the-counter.

Brain Fatigue Preventive Measures

Brain fatigue is often a controllable condition, if one is able to determine the underlying cause of it. Some activities that may help reduce the episodes of brain fatigue include:

- ✤ **SLEEP**: Eight hours of uninterrupted sleep has been shown to provide the best rejuvenating benefits. Try to increase the quality of your sleep to help reduce brain fatigue during the day. For my best tips to sleep like a baby night after night, please refer to my book *Choose to Thrive*.

- **QUIT SMOKING AND/OR ALCOHOL**: Smoking and alcohol dramatically increase the number of free radicals being produced in the body, and this can play a role in mental confusion and poor brain health. Limiting intake of both will allow your body's antioxidants to start the healing process immediately.

- **EAT A HEALTHIER DIET**: A diet with plenty of fresh whole foods rich in omega-3, -6 and -9 fatty acids, magnesium, and B complex vitamins will help reduce the episodes of brain fatigue.

- **REDUCE STRESS**: Stress can literally be a killer, so practicing ways to reduce stress in your daily life can be quite helpful. Whether through exercise, meditation, mindful deep breathing, or another calming practice, reducing stress will help alleviate brain fog and help you to live a healthier life. Sounds of nature are very calming. To enjoy these sounds of nature in the comfort of your home or office or anywhere/anytime, please refer to my website SusanSmithJones.com

- **EXERCISE**: It's been known for some time that exercise can lift your mood, ward off depression, and help the brain age more gracefully—free of memory loss and dementia. And now researchers have found that even just one bout of exercise can—even better than a cup of coffee—improve your mental focus and cognitive performance for any challenging task you face that day. A new analysis of 19 studies published in the *British Medical Journal* found that short 10 to 40 minute bursts of exercise led to an immediate boost in concentration and mental focus, improving blood flow to the brain.

- **INCREASE ANTIOXIDANT INTAKE**: Eating a healthy diet naturally increases one's antioxidants. These powerful and healing substances, which are predominantly found in the fresh fruits and vegetables we eat, prohibit (and in many cases prevent) the oxidation of other molecules in the body.

- **MOLECULAR HYDROGEN THERAPY**: Molecular hydrogen, my favorite support for the brain along with sleep, is proven to improve memory and cognitive function by alleviating the damage caused by oxidative stress, but its effects go much further than that. Diseases and conditions such as Parkinson's, Alzheimer's, TBI (traumatic brain injury), hemorrhagic stroke, and ischemic brain injury are all positively affected by hydrogen therapy. Hydrogen can also offer preventive measures against these and other brain disorders due to its size, its ability to pass the blood/brain barrier, and its antioxidant properties. So . . . don't forget to take your hydrogen!

I take it daily in the forms of a simple tablet and also use an inhaler, and I also use a mister on my face and neck with hydrogen water to help keep my skin youthful. Visit SusanSmithJones.com and go to "Favorite Products" in the navigation bar and then scroll down to the many articles I have posted on Molecular Hydrogen and how it supports high-level wellness. You'll find countless, enthralling scientific studies supporting Molecular Hydrogen Therapy that will captivate you, too. Additionally, you will also find the very best place to get the tablets (High Tech Health in Boulder, CO—see below for the telephone number) that dissolve in water and the Molecular Hydrogen Inhaler, the same ones that I use and highly recommend, and also how **to get the same discount that I get using the code SUSAN10.** (To call the company and ask questions, contact: **800-794-5355 (USA & Canada) or 303-413-8500 (International).**

I wouldn't be without either the Molecular Hydrogen Inhaler or Tablets; they are definitely front and center in my healthy living program. I use the inhaler when working at my desk, watching television, or reading. I even take it with me when traveling since it only weighs a few pounds and is portable. In fact, I am using it right now as I am writing this book to help keep my brain sharp and focused. It really works and is so valuable for vitality.

It is not an overestimate to say that hydrogen's
impact on therapeutic and preventative
medicine could be enormous in the future.

~Free Radical Research 2010

HOW TO STRENGTHEN YOUR BRAIN . . .
AT ANY AGE

To support your goal of having a fit brain at any age, you need to adhere to two basic principles: variety and curiosity. When any activity becomes second nature to you, you want to move in the direction of more brain stimulation. For example, if you always create the same recipes in your kitchen for your family, move out of your familiar box and try some new and more complicated recipes. If your crossword puzzles no longer challenge you and you can do them in your sleep, you'll want to progress to something more demanding. Your goal is to move on to a new challenge to get the best workout for your brain.

Additionally, in your quest for mental fitness, keep a keen, wide-eyed curiosity about the world around you, how it works, and how you can understand it all. Young children are naturally this way. They are often enthralled by everything, including doing dishes, vacuuming, watering the plants, and watching butterflies and other insects. Being captivated and amazed by your environment is easy to do when you are able to travel to different locations in your community, country, and worldwide to enjoy different cultures, languages, sights, smells, and surroundings. If you are not able to travel, then here's a tip for you: Peruse travel books and magazines or watch television programs about traveling to different locations in the world to stimulate your brain. Then write down a dozen things you enjoyed about the program or travel magazine that fascinated you. Next, by telephone or in person, tell someone else why you enjoyed the information you learned and relate as many details as possible. In other words, keeping your brain working fast and efficiently is like doing cardio exercises for your brain muscles. Make as one of your health goals to continue teasing and challenging your brain.

As mentioned in the chapters on meditation, choosing to meditate each day will stimulate your brain in a very positive way. In fact, it's one of the best things you can do to work out your brain's muscles, according to scientific studies. Yes, meditation relaxes you, but at the same time, it also gives your brain a workout by creating a different mental state in which your brain activity changes. When your meditation time is over, you feel refreshed, reinvigorated, confident, and hopeful. It's an unbeatable combination to infuse your day with more enlivenment — especially if you choose to meditate early morning. What a great way to start off your day on a positive note!

Tips for Strengthening the Mind through Brain Fitness and Training

To reiterate, exercise plays an important role in one's health and wellness, and while often forgotten, it absolutely applies to the brain. When the brain is exercised, it helps prevent depreciation of one's mental faculties as they age. Like any other muscle in the body, the brain can be strengthened through the implementation of regular brain exercise.

BRAIN EXERCISES FOR MEMORY: Memory is often one of the first things to go as we age, and this can be truly debilitating because memory plays a key role in all of our cognitive abilities. Exercises to help improve memory can consist of listening to a song you've never heard and trying to memorize the lyrics, playing games designed to help you focus on your recall abilities, taking a shower or getting dressed in the dark, or learning a second language.

You can also practice visual-spatial cognitive function by walking into a room and focusing on five objects, and then leaving the room and trying to recall what the objects were and where they were located in the room. Try to recall the objects and their locations again in two hours. If this proves to be too easy, then increase the difficulty by trying to recall details such as the color of the items, the direction they are pointing, or other minor details.

BRAIN EXERCISES FOR COMPREHENSION: Learning new words is a great way to increase one's vocabulary, improve grammar, and grow mental comprehension. After perusing Chapter 1, you can see why I am very partial to this brain exercise tip—being a logophile, of course! A great way to exercise the brain to improve comprehension is to expose your brain to words you may not be familiar with. You can do this by reading a section of the newspaper you regularly avoid or by reading a book in a genre you haven't tried before. By doing this, chances are you will find a wide array of words that you have never seen before and common words used in ways you never thought of. To find all of my 260 positive words that bring me great joy to use often, please refer to SusanSmithJones. com and put in the search bar "260 Positive Words" and you'll find my favorites to help you speak and write in a more positive light.

BRAIN EXERCISES FOR IMPROVING FOCUS: A good attention span is critical in today's world where distractions are found at every corner. Performing mental exercises to enhance concentration will help keep your brain focused at all times. A good exercise to help improve attention and focus is doing two things at once, like listening to an audiobook while doing the dishes or doing math in your head while taking a shower.

BRAIN EXERCISES FOR EXECUTIVE FUNCTION: Executive function is our ability to solve problems using reasoning and logic. A good way to exercise this ability is to play games that require you to make quick decisions. There are many games out there, both digital and analog, that can be a lot of fun to play.

Transcend Infrared Sauna

Infrared saunas have been shown to improve vascular function, blood pressure, reduce inflammation, and boost cognition. One study found that Finnish men who frequently used saunas had a significant reduction in dementia and Alzheimer's risk. With Alzheimer's disease now clocking in as the third most common cause of death in the United States, any technique that can help resist the impacts of dementia onset adds hope. Visit my website to find out more about the Transcend Infrared Sauna, why I wouldn't be without my home's personal sauna, and where to purchase one at a discount. For now, you can all the company High Tech Health that makes the best infrared saunas in the industry and where I purchased mine. To call with questions or to order, contact: **800-794-5355 (USA & Canada) or 303-413-8500 (International).**

Choose today to start taking better care of your brain.

Therefore if any man be in Christ, he is a new creature:
old things are passed away; behold, all things become new.

~2 Corinthians 5:17

The idea is to write it so that people hear it and it slides
through the brain and goes straight to the heart.

~Maya Angelou

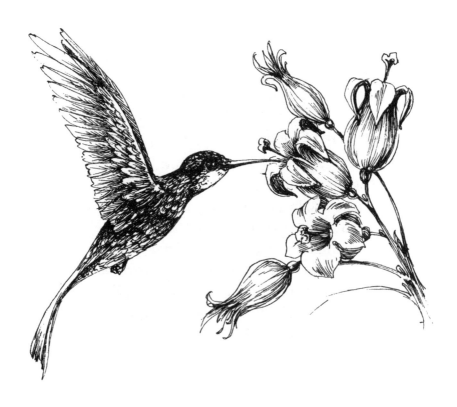

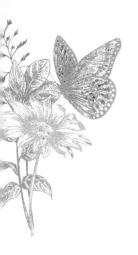

Chapter 4

Choosing Foods for Brain Vitality

Books, the children of the brain.

~Jonathan Swift

The brain is a wonderful organ; it starts working the moment you get up in the morning and does not stop until you get into the office.

~Robert Frost

While we might not be able to be in control of all aspects concerning our personal brain health since genetics are involved, we can certainly choose which foods to eat and which to eschew to help maximize our brains' abilities well into old age. It's been well established, also, in recent decades that the brain and gut are related, the gut often being referred to as a "second brain" or a second nervous system. Although it's not the same as the brain in that it doesn't "think," it does have 100 billion neurons, and, therefore, like the brain, determines our mood. So it's not just our physical health that foods affect but our mental and emotional health as well. Here are some of the foods to avoid and some to include in your diet to support high-level brain function.

Foods to Avoid

GLUTEN: Gluten is not a food but a composite of proteins found in wheat, grains, barley, and corn. Gluten is no stranger to controversy, and its declining reputation over the last decade or so is for good reason.

Wheat is an ancient food and a dietary staple of many cultures. But our modern iteration is a different version of the food that sustained our ancestors. This is due to modern milling practices, genetic modification, and the added sugar. Today, the number of people diagnosed with celiac disease is four times higher than it was just fifty years ago. And more people than ever are suffering gluten sensitivity. It's pretty clear that food conglomerates, in the name of efficiency and cutting costs, have corrupted what was once a primary food source.

So no, it's no secret anymore that gluten is the culprit in many unhappy digestive tracts, but gluten is also associated with many mental disorders, including anxiety, depression, emotional disorders, and even schizophrenia. In some studies, doctors treating schizophrenics alleviated symptoms by eliminating gluten in patients' diets. The same is true for patients with depression, anxiety, and manic depressive disorders. What's interesting is that the study's patients did not necessarily suffer from celiac disease. Researchers hypothesize that gluten is a virulent property, and when eliminated from the diet, mental health issues can be mitigated. This is promising news for many suffering from organic brain disorders and chemical imbalances.

DAIRY: Inflammation is the underlying cause of many physical disorders and diseases, but it is also the underlying cause of many emotional disorders as well, and casein is quite well known for its relationship to inflammation. In dairy's case, the culprit is casein. This is the protein found in milk and it has, like gluten, been similarly linked to schizophrenia, bipolar disorder, depression, and even psychosis. But even if it doesn't lead to a severe emotional disorder, it still may be impacting your mood, as it's been linked to anger, aggression, and irritability. Studies seem to be also indicating a link to autism. And autism-related aggression is often reduced when dairy is eliminated from the diet of sufferers. And diets high in dairy sometimes create bipolar-related behaviors in those without bipolar disorder. Anecdotally, I have observed many friends' and clients' lives transform after I've advised them to eliminate dairy (and gluten) to improve their moods and emotional disorders.

Many have noted such a significant improvement that they were able to give up their antidepressants altogether and control their symptoms naturally.

WHITE SUGAR: We already know that we're not doing our body any favors by consuming white sugar. But your brain won't be congratulating you on your sugary food choices either, even though its reward center may simultaneously be coaxing you to indulge. Yes, sugary food is tasty and often shared at birthday parties and other celebratory and holiday events. But what it does to your brain is nothing to celebrate. High sugar intake can affect mood, memory, and a host of other cognitive functions. Studies link it to lower test scores. And if those aren't compelling enough reasons, high sugar consumption is also related to brain shrinkage, dementia, and even Alzheimer's disease. Avoid cakes, cookies, and all the usual suspects, but remember that it often shows up in ostensibly healthy options like fruit drinks and packaged fruit snacks.

WHITE FLOUR AND REFINED CARBOHYDRATES: The flour lurking in many tasty but sabotaging foods like pasta, cakes, chips, muffins, pizza, etc. as well as in potatoes, white rice, and sweetened sodas, among many others, is no friend to your waistline. But it's also out to sabotage your cognitive abilities as well, namely your memory. Too many refined carbohydrates in the system cause a high glycemic index, which spikes insulin. This leads to inflammation, which can thus lead to memory loss. *It only takes one meal to observe the change according to studies!* Extended consumption can impair the memory in much more serious ways by leading to dementia and Alzheimer's disease. Refined carb consumption has also been linked to depression in postmenopausal women.

ASPARTAME: One of the ingredients in the artificial sweetener is something that may impede the production of neurotransmitters. The studies on this product are less conclusive, but some research has shown that aspartame can markedly affect mood, causing irritability. Additionally, it has been found to impair cognitive functioning on mental acuity tests as well as being linked to strokes, depression, and like most of the other items on this list, dementia.

FISH CONTAINING HIGH LEVELS OF MERCURY: Fish is a source of protein and other minerals, including omega-3's, and is recommended by some health professionals as part of a healthy diet. Certain fish, however, should be consumed only in moderation if at all because of their high mercury content, which undermines the point of eating fish. The fish on that list include shark, tuna, mackerel, orange roughy, and tilefish. The high levels of mercury have even more serious implications for the brain than some of the other foods on this list because mercury is toxic and will not only disrupt the formation of neurotransmitters but can also damage the central nervous system and thus the brain through the neurotoxins, which release the toxic mercury. Especially susceptible to these effects are unborn fetuses and children. Some experts advise only eating the fish on this list once or twice a week, but I recommend avoiding these fish altogether to prevent any disruption to our brain's functioning—especially since there are so many other healthy options from which to choose.

HIGHLY PROCESSED FOODS: These are the foods which you already know to be unhealthy but perhaps can't help but indulge in anyway. Sometimes it's out of convenience, like with ready-made prepackaged meals, or out of a need to indulge in something salty, like we do at times with comfort foods. These foods include microwaveable pizza, microwave popcorn, ketchup, instant noodles, chips, etc. Most of us know that the added fats, sugar, and salt in these foods are the enemy of bathing suit season, but they may also be contributing to decreased cognitive functioning. There are implications for brain plasticity, according to studies, in addition to impaired ability to reason or perform on cognitive tests. These foods can even lead to a decrease in brain tissue, which is a cause of Alzheimer's disease. They also disrupt what is known as the blood-brain barrier, which protects the brain by preventing damaging substances from entering. When this is disrupted because of highly processed foods, long-term memory is affected.

TRANS FATS: Foods high in trans fats are also enemies of the brain and body—so much so that the FDA banned them in 2018. However, products made before June 2018 can still be sold. And other companies are still slipping them into their products by using trace amounts, which however small, are still harmful. The effects include the standard list: memory loss, a decline in cognitive functioning, lower brain volume, and Alzheimer's disease. The foods that still contain some trans fats are often listed in the ingredients as partially hydrogenated oil. Check the labels of the following foods: margarine, vegetable oils, vegetable shortening, and nondairy coffee creamer. And an honorable mention goes to microwave popcorn and bakery products for showing up a second time on our list (microwave popcorn is also highly processed and bakery products also contain gluten).

ALCOHOL: This last one should come as no surprise since the changes to the brain are immediate and often even the desired effect. However, the effects of long-term usage are a good deal less desirable. A deficiency in vitamin B1 is often a consequence of alcoholism and can lead to several diseases such as Korsakoff syndrome or Wernicke encephalopathy. The brain-related damage associated with these diseases are confusion, memory loss, lack of equilibrium, and even problems with eyesight. But even just one night out on the town can be problematic if you're binge drinking because the temporary brain-related damage can cause a drinker to make bad choices and put him or herself in harm's way. This could end up causing even more brain-related damage if you're in a head-on collision while drinking and driving, not to mention the fights and other skirmishes people so often find themselves in when binge drinking. Take heart though, as there is still a smattering of health-related benefits with low alcohol consumption such as in red wine. The antioxidant, resveratrol, is in grapes, supplements, and other foods. The resveratrol in red wine comes from the skin of grapes used to make wine. Because red wine is fermented with grape skins longer than is white wine, red wine contains more resveratrol. While I choose not to drink any alcohol at all (and if I did, I would opt for organic red or white wines), if you do imbibe, please always drink moderately and responsibly.

Foods to Feed Your Brain

NUTS AND SEEDS: Vitamin E is the secret ingredient in these delicious snacks and/or garnishes. Vitamin E is known to reduce general cognitive decline as we age. But one nut in particular stands out for both its vitamin E as well as the ALA (alpha-linolenic acid) it contains. ALA is an omega-3 fatty acid which is linked to better heart health because it improves blood flow, the same reason it positively impacts the brain. It begins with the letter "W"—can you guess what it is? In studies, participants consuming higher amounts of delicious and versatile walnuts performed better on cognitive tests. What a tasty way to improve your mind.

BERRIES: These delicious little fruits are loaded with flavonoids, which are associated in studies with improved memory. Due to an ability to ward against oxidative stress in the brain, in animal studies, they have been shown to decrease the effects associated with dementia and Alzheimer's disease. Berries are a delicious way to make the brain more resilient. And more specifically, of all the berries, blueberries are the most powerful berry and have the nickname of the "brain berry." They are loaded with antioxidants, which can protect the brain from free radical damage and promote healthy brain aging.

FATTY FISH: These are also abundant in omega-3 fatty acids, which, as we already know, is good for our brains. Beta-amyloid is a protein buildup in Alzheimer's sufferers and the fatty acids in omega-3's also help to lower these damaging clumps. It's important though to choose fish that are not high in mercury since that will not only undermine the positive effects of the fatty acids but will increase the likelihood of damaging neurotransmitters. Fish to choose from are salmon, cod, herring, sardines, pollack, and light canned tuna.

AVOCADOS: Once eschewed for their high-fat content, avocados are now darlings of the health food world. And what they've done for bread is no small feat, bringing it back from exile and helping it rebrand as "healthy," when in the form of avocado toast. Besides all of the nutrients it floods our bodies with, it is also a terrific food to add to the list of brain foods. The healthy unsaturated fats in these guys help improve blood flow to the brain, which can reduce oxidative stress. We already know from the earlier discussion that oxidative stress is a factor in dementia and Alzheimer's disease. Furthermore, avocados helped to prevent nerve damage in the brains of animals when they were exposed to low oxygen. This has implications for the prefrontal cortex, which is the part of the brain responsible for critical thinking. So enjoy an avocado, but if it's avocado toast, make sure the bread is gluten free, since gluten is on the brain food "naughty list."

LEAFY GREENS: Lutein, vitamin K, folate, and beta-carotene are a few of the nutrients in these well-known-for-their-health-benefits foods. Eleven years younger is how much participants in studies seemed compared to their peers in term of cognitive decline. One cup daily is all it takes. A study in which the average age of the participants was 81 was conducted over 5 years. The ones who ate the most leafy greens had the lowest rate of cognitive decline. Specifically, leafy greens help with episodic memory, working memory, semantic memory, visuospatial ability, and perceptual speed. And a diet high in leafy greens seems to reduce the risk of Alzheimer's disease by up to 53%. That is not insignificant. So break out that spinach, kale, lettuce, romaine lettuce, Swiss chard, sprouts, and collards. Even if you're not a senior, it's never too early to start preventing cognitive decline.

TURMERIC: Remember the beta-amyloids discussed earlier in "Fatty Fish"? It's the protein buildup, or plaque, that contributes to Alzheimer's disease. The omega-3's are a sort of Drano for the brain, dissolving the plaque. Well, the curcumin in turmeric is another property that helps to clear away these toxic proteins and protect against Alzheimer's disease in addition to alleviating symptoms for those who already suffer from it. Turmeric is a main ingredient in curry, an Indian spice showing up in many Indian dishes. And guess what? The prevalence of Alzheimer's disease in India is 4 to 5 times less than it is in America. And guess what else? Indian food is delicious. So start cooking with this ingredient today—or if curries aren't your thing, take turmeric supplements, which are widely available these days. You'll also help your memory and even mood since studies have linked turmeric to improvements in those areas as well. I stir a teaspoon of organic turmeric powder into my large glass of alkaline water with lemon every morning.

DARK CHOCOLATE: Not many people are going to complain about having to try to accommodate this into their diets. This is probably the most delicious way to help improve your brain's health. Since it improves blood flow to the brain, it can help produce many desirable effects including general cognitive functioning in the elderly and can improve verbal fluency in everyone! It's also been proven to prevent age-related memory decline and improve neuroplasticity, memory, and even mood. Personally, I find that sometimes all I need to do is think about eating dark chocolate to experience a mood boost!

BLACK & GREEN TEA: The flavonoids in these teas are also the properties in berries and dark chocolate. Flavonoids are antioxidants. But green and black tea are also full of many other types of antioxidants as well. All of these help to reduce that pesky oxidative stress that we've been discussing that erodes brain function. Not only that, but by blocking adenosine, caffeine increases the amount of neurotransmitters firing in the brain. You've heard of dopamine, right? Well that's one of the neurotransmitters released and it's a mood elevator. Caffeine also increases reaction time and improves memory and is associated with higher cognitive functioning on tests. But it's the added component of L-theanine that exists in these teas that, in conjunction with caffeine, works to increase alpha-waves and dopamine in the brain, again, associated with good moods and even anxiety reduction.

WATER: Our brain cells rely on water to operate. When they're not hydrated, concentration and focus can become issues, which is something you're probably aware of from experience. Insufficient amounts in the cells also will hinder both short- and long-term memory. Water also removes toxins from the body, toxins that could otherwise end up affecting the brain. It also optimizes blood flow, which is necessary to stabilize mood and for a good night sleep. General mental fatigue, confusion, and even headaches also often result from a lack of hydration. And finally, and most surprisingly, staying hydrated can even help with anxiety. Don't just wait for your body to signal to you that you're thirsty. Act preemptively and keep drinking all day. You optimize your physical abilities too when you do! As mentioned previously, I have been using an Ionizer Plus device from High Tech Health for over 20 years to make delicious, purified alkaline water. Under "Favorite Products" on my website, you will find several articles about the healing power and benefits of drinking alkaline water—my beverage of choice. To ask questions or order this same machine for your kitchen that I have, contact High Tech Health in Boulder, CO, at: **800-794-5355 (USA & Canada) or 303-413-8500 (International)**

CITRUS FRUITS: These zesty treats have the ability to lower your risks of dementia by 23%. Those are not bad odds. And the flavonoids in these fruits can ward off other neurodegenerative diseases like Parkinson's and Alzheimer's disease. These specific flavonoids also have the ability to protect brain cells, which has a number of implications for the brain's overall health.

EGGS: The choline in eggs helps to strengthen memory and improve mood. But it's more than choline that qualifies eggs for this list. It's their profusion of B vitamins, something very important for brain health since they decrease the rate of mental decline in the elderly. Folate and B12, something eggs are in high supply of, are often lacking in those with depression. Many doctors in recent years have discovered that patients who adjust their diets to include more B vitamins, and/or who add supplements, are able to address their depression without pharmaceuticals.

If you eat a plant-based diet and want to increase your choline intake, as I strive to do, your most nutrient-rich options include collard greens, Brussels sprouts, broccoli, Swiss chard, cauliflower, and asparagus.

GARLIC: Garlic makes the brain happy—literally. It is a natural serotonin booster. And I'm not saying that you should indulge in smoking and heavy drinking, but if you do, garlic is actually filled with enough of something called FruArg (a carbohydrate derivative that promotes the production of antioxidants to the brain cells), which can fortify your brain against these and other environmental stressors. It actually will help to rebuild damaged brain cells. Garlic also produces a lot of the ever important nitric oxide in the brain, which is necessary also to fight off, again, dementia and Alzheimer's disease. In short, garlic is not called a "superfood" for no reason.

It seems very clear: many foods can make your mind feel unclear. You may have been avoiding many of the foods on the so-called "naughty list" because of what we know about their power to harm our bodies. But now we know how important it is to avoid them for our cognitive health as well. It's important to remember, too, how inextricably linked our bodies and brains actually are and that the gut is indeed the "second brain." Mental disturbances affect the way we feel physically and vice versa. The good news is that we have the power to determine so much about how we feel and even about how we age by making the right food choices. Knowledge is power. And this new knowledge goes even further by helping our minds stay supple and young into old age.

There is a real danger that computers will develop
intelligence and take over. We urgently need to develop
direct connections to the brain so that computers can add
to human intelligence rather than be in opposition.

~STEPHEN HAWKING

A fool's brain digests philosophy into folly,
science into superstition, and art into pedantry.
Hence University education.

~GEORGE BERNARD SHAW

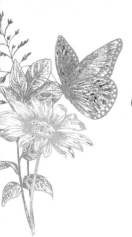

Chapter 5

Cleansing & Detoxifying
Head-to-Toe

The doctor of the future will no longer treat
the human frame with drugs, but rather will
cure and prevent disease with nutrition.

~Thomas Edison

There is absolutely no substitute for greens in the diet!
If you refuse to eat these 'sunlight energy' foods,
you are depriving yourself, to a large degree,
of the very essence of life.

~H. E. Kirschner, MD

We are not separate from our environment. As our environment becomes increasingly polluted, the toxic burden on our bodies increases as well. Heavy metals, pesticides, and other toxins can interfere with our hormones, affect our gut health, and accumulate in our bodies, leading to health problems like allergies, autoimmune disease, cancer, obesity, and more.

Supporting our detoxification systems, like our liver and digestion, is essential to health optimization and disease prevention. Eating organic foods, testing for heavy metals, and incorporating targeted supplements and therapies, like molecular hydrogen, alkaline water, and infrared saunas, are powerful ways to reduce toxic exposure and boost the body's ability to eliminate these harmful substances. So are you ready to bolster your body's detoxification and rejuvenation systems?

Anytime of the year is a perfect time of year to embark on a detox/ cleanse program. In case you're not aware, there is an epidemic sweeping America and the UK that I refer to as "internal toxic pollution." Many people suffer from chronic disease and loss of health not only as a direct result of unhealthy conditions environmentally, but internally as well—within the human body. We often think of health as the absence of disease. But is this truly health? Are we healthy one day and then all of a sudden sick the next? There's a plethora of evidence that demonstrates to us that health or sickness is a process that develops over a period of time (often years) and is based at the cellular level.

Our bodies are made of over 70 trillion cells. Cells of the same ilk join together to form organs, tissue, bones, blood, etc. Each cell is constantly in the process of dying and being replaced. Each cell receives nutrition and expels waste and toxins, which must be eliminated from the body in a timely manner. When the cells are deficient in nutrients or are overpowered with toxins and waste, cellular malfunction begins and thus the slow decline in the level of health until one day a disease state is recognized by the manifestation of symptoms.

There are thousands of toxic chemicals all around us. There are pesticides in our foods, chemicals in our water, and pollutants in the air we breathe. Even common cosmetics are full of chemicals. We drink, eat, breathe, and live in a soup of toxic chemicals. One of the greatest health secrets is that you have control over the pollution in your body. If you keep a balanced and clean internal environment, you won't succumb to the toxic buildup so prevalent in most people's bodies. *Those who cleanse regularly look and feel younger, are much healthier, and live a longer life than those who ignore the need to internally cleanse.*

Are You Toxic?

The following are some of the possible symptoms of toxic buildup in the body: constipation; chronic yeast infections; brittle hand and toe nails; frequent colds; weight gain or difficulty in losing weight; acne, dry or pale skin; mood swings or depression; low sex drive; lack of concentration; feckless short-term memory; sleeping problems; frequent headaches; chronic urinary tract infections; arthritic bone pains or rheumatism; allergies, gas, bloating, flatulence; general weakness; and frequent/chronic fatigue or lack of energy, just to name a few.

Our modern diets are to blame for many of our most common ailments. Many people are digging their graves with their knives and forks and are making life-and-death decisions every time they sit down to a meal or snack. Disease often occurs as a result of an unhealthy lifestyle, which causes the body to become sluggish, congested, acidic, and polluted. Antibiotics, excess sugar, carbonated beverages, chemical food additives, and over-the-counter drugs can alter the acid/alkaline balance of the intestinal tract, often killing beneficial bacteria and creating the perfect environment for harmful microbes to grow. Without the "good" or "friendly" bacteria to keep them in check, these "bad" bacteria can eventually overrun our body and severely depress our immune system.

Mucoid plaque is a slimy gel-like substance that covers the inner lining of the intestines and bowel. Plaque harbors toxins and interferes with nutrient absorption. The colon is known to hold up to 30 or more pounds of old matter and can be packed with undigested foods and disease-promoting bacteria.

Additionally, parasites are a toxic menace and can wreak havoc in your body. When faulty digestion keeps food from being properly processed and sent out of the body, undigested food can remain in the body and create fermentation and putrefaction. This can cause parasites and germ life to develop. Parasites thrive in an unhealthy, unclean colon. When the bowel contains partially digested proteins, sugars, or starches, it can harbor an alarming variety of parasites. These parasites can range from microscopic organisms to tapeworms 15 inches long.

Benefits of Cleansing

So what can internal cleansing do for you? Here are some of the most commonly reported benefits of cleansing and detoxifying the body: relief from bloating; flatter abdominal area; relief from constipation; clearer thinking; greater sense of well-being; stronger immune system; improved digestion; better sleep; youthful appearance and healthier skin; and more energy and confidence! Simply put, internal cleansing can dramatically improve the quality of your overall health. It's also one of the best ways to break any bad food habits you might have such as always salting foods, being addicted to white sugar/white flour products and sodas, etc.

When the colon and liver are clear of excess toxins and waste, it frees up energy to be used by the rest of the body. It also helps the liver and intestinal tract to manufacture nutrients as well as absorb them from your food much more efficiently. This supports the healing, repair, and maintenance of your entire body.

When to Cleanse and What to Expect

During these past four decades, I have embraced the following cleansing schedule: One day a week, 2 to 3 days monthly, 7 to 10 days with each change of season, and 30 to 40 days every two to three years, I engage in some kind of detox/cleanse program to preclude a toxic buildup in my body and to keep me vibrantly healthy. In addition, for over 30 years I have also created custom-designed cleanses and health programs for my clients worldwide, depending on their personal needs. In other words, I'm passionate about the healing power of whole-body cleansing.

Depending on how toxic your body may be, and how long you choose to cleanse, during your detox, you may feel a bit more tired than usual. If that's the case, just make sure to get more rest. Some people report feeling more energy; others have broken out with rashes on the skin, but these go away in a few days; some experience a slight fever or headaches (that's a sign that your body is housecleaning); most people release lots of mucus during the cleanse; others experience mood swings or depression. At the end of a detox program, most will feel "lighter" and more peaceful; certainly you'll feel in more control over your body and experience an increase in self-esteem and confidence.

The Body's Largest Organ – Your Skin

Weighing in at approximately six pounds and covering an area of about two square yards, your skin is the largest organ of the body. Not only is it an organ, but the skin is also a major area for the elimination of toxic wastes from our systems. It has been called our "third kidney" because it works closely with the kidneys to help release uric acid. Our body must eliminate large amounts of waste products from our systems daily or we will die. The bowel, lungs, kidneys, and skin are our four channels of elimination. Each of these organs ideally should release two pounds of toxins per day. Therefore, our skin is responsible for getting rid of nearly a fourth of our bodily toxins each and every day. If the skin is not doing its job, the kidneys, lungs, and bowel will have an extra load with which to deal.

Skin brushing is one of the finest ways to detoxify the skin and promote good circulation. While I discuss the healing power of dry skin brushing (as well as detoxification and cleansing) in my book *Body Temple Vitality*, here's a brief summary. Make a commitment for 30 days of dry skin brushing. After one month, your skin will feel and look about 10 years younger with daily dry skin brushing. Your brush should be made from natural vegetable fibers, not nylon or other synthetic material. Brush your entire body (except your face and private areas) *before* you shower or bathe. Brushing the skin dry rather than wet is very important because it does a much better job of removing dead skin cells and toxins. I use a special smaller, softer brush for my face and neck.

Infrared Sauna

If you do a quick Google search, you'll find a lot of people knocking the ability of saunas to flush toxins, but we've known for a long time that sweating helps the body rid itself of toxins. As mentioned earlier, your skin is your biggest organ of elimination.

Studies have found that increased sweating, as experienced in a sauna, can help you excrete toxic metals like arsenic, cadmium, lead, and mercury. One study found "that body stores of trace metals may be depleted during prolonged exposure to heat."

Another study found that "induced sweating in saunas can mobilize BPA in adipose tissue thus leading to enhanced excretion in sweat."

The science is there—sweating helps you eliminate toxins and infrared saunas can help you sweat at a much faster rate and are much comfortable for relaxation because they don't feel as suffocatingly hot as traditional dry saunas.

If you want to know the difference of a dry sauna or a wet/stream sauna, please visit my website, SusanSmithJones.com, and in the search bar, put in the words "Dry vs Wet Sauna" and you can read my article and learn much more about *Heat Therapy: Sweating Your Way to Vitality.* I highly recommend getting an infrared sauna for your home. They come in different sizes to fit even the smallest space constraints. Under "Favorite Products" on my website, find the article titled "10 Benefits of Infrared Sauna Therapy." For now, you can call the company High Tech Health **(800-794-5355 or 303-413-8500** or visit HighTechHealth. com) that makes the best infrared saunas in the industry and where I purchased mine. Ask them any questions you might have or how to get a substantial discount on your purchase (using my name "SSJ") on a one-, two-, or three-person Transcend Infrared Sauna. Remember, the gift of health is the best gift you can give yourself.

Your Personal Cleanse

There are many aspects to internal cleansing that are too numerous to mention in this chapter so here's a brief summary. Whether it's a 1-Day or 30-Day Cleanse, here are many of the things I embrace as part of my cleansing program. See how many you can incorporate into your program. You can find more detailed information on everything mentioned below in my books *Choose to Thrive, The Curative Kitchen & Lifestyle,* and *Kitchen Gardening.*

1. **PLANT-BASED FOOD & FRESH JUICES:** Foods can heal. I am sure that you have noticed that when you eat better, you feel better. It's not complicated. While on a cleanse, adopt a plant-based diet with as many raw or "living" foods as possible. I also drink organic detox teas that I purchase from my local health food store or from Penn Herb Company. High water content foods—especially fresh fruit and vegetables—are

easy to digest. Emphasize any leafy greens because the greens are very detoxifying and rejuvenating. As my grandmother always used to say to me, "When you are green inside, you are clean inside." These fresh, colorful foods take stress off of your digestive system. For short cleansing programs, you may want to consume only raw food or just drink fresh vegetable juices. Consider one day a week consuming delicious green smoothies. (In Chapter 17, you will find lots of wonderful recipes the entire family will love.) Also, everyone should have a good home juicer so you can make fresh juices. Refer to Chapter 14 for more information on the benefits of fresh vegetable juices and raw foods.

2. NETI NASAL CLEANSING: The practice of nasal irrigation, known as Neti, has been used by practitioners of Ayurveda in India for thousands of years. Many people in America practice Neti on a daily basis to keep their sinuses clean and improve their ability to breathe freely. Most find it a soothing and pleasant practice once they try it. Dr. Oz has discussed the benefits of nasal cleansing a few times. Why cleanse your body and ignore your nasal passages? There are many videos online to show you how to do this.

3. SUNSHINE & AIR: Enjoy approximately 10 to 20 minutes of healing sunshine on as much of your body's skin as possible; avoid the midday sun. During your cleanse, breathe in fresh, clean air. This is the perfect time to do your deep breathing practice several times each day. Additionally, walk barefoot on the grass, in your garden, or on the sand at the beach. This is called grounding or earthing. This will help keep your body detoxified. Even 5 to 10 minutes will make a positive difference. Refer to page 219 in Chapter 14 to learn about earthing or how to get a simple mat for your feet to use at home that will give you the same benefits as going outdoors. I put my earthing mat under my desk and am using it as I am writing this book. Also, please visit my website, and under "Favorite Products," read the article I wrote on earthing and watch the amazing, short documentary I posted to teach you about this healthful practice.

4. WATER: Drink at least eight glasses of purified water daily (preferably alkaline water from the **Ionizer Plus** devise discussed earlier), between meals. When your body is fully hydrated, you can more easily flush toxins out of your system. Keeping the body hydrated with fresh water takes stress off of the liver and the colon, two of the body's channels of elimination.

5. MEDITATE & REST: Find time for quiet reflection and relaxation during your detoxification program. This is not the time to fill your life with unlimited activity. Instead, choose to slow down, smell the flowers, keep a gratitude journal, and simplify your life.

6. SIMPLIFY & READ: When I'm doing a cleanse, long or short, I will often find simple ways to declutter my surroundings. In other words, I cleanse my body, soul, and environment. This is also an excellent time to read books on how to take better care of your body. Any of my books are perfect to read, including *Choose to Thrive* and *Be the Change.* My favorite thing to read when doing a cleanse is the Bible because it inspires my mind and heart as I am physically nurturing my body.

7. EXERCISE: It's important to work out during a cleanse. If you're feeling tired, do some yoga stretches or other simple movements. Make sure to include aerobic activity such as walking to help with your circulation. For detailed info on all aspects of exercise and how to stay motivated to your program, please refer to my book *Invest in Yourself with Exercise.*

8. HOT BATHS & MASSAGE: A hot bath is also an excellent way to facilitate the removal of toxins through the skin. To make the bath more relaxing, use the essential oil of lavender, which has been proven to promote relaxation and tranquility. Also, during a cleanse, schedule in time to get a massage. If possible, find a massage therapist who knows how to do a lymph massage, which will also help flush the toxins out of your body.

9. BUDDY CLEANSE: Sometimes I'll find a friend who will do the cleanse with me. Even though we might both live in different homes, or even across the country or world, it is still comforting to know that there's someone else (friend or family) joining you on the cleanse. Each day, visit with that person, even if it's over the telephone or by email/text, and compare notes and encourage each other on.

Keep in mind that the secret to vibrant health, youth, and vitality is in cleansing the body and mind and then adopting a lifestyle that includes positive, grateful thoughts, natural foods, pure water, fresh air, sunshine, and exercise. Learning to cleanse the body and mind is an essential part of healing. When the body is burdened with toxic waste material, it will be tired and have low immune function. When the body is clean, it can absorb the essential nutrients it needs to heal, repair, and maintain good health. So the next time you hear the expression, "Cleanliness is next to godliness," you may understand better that it conveys an extremely important aspect of health and rejuvenation. The more cleansed you keep your miraculous body, the more room you'll have to be filled with Light.

The wise man should consider that health
is the greatest of human blessings.

~HIPPOCRATES

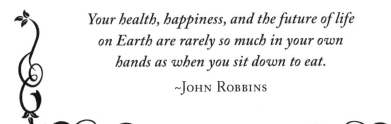

Your health, happiness, and the future of life
on Earth are rarely so much in your own
hands as when you sit down to eat.

~JOHN ROBBINS

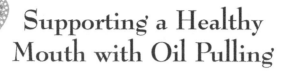

Chapter 6

Supporting a Healthy Mouth with Oil Pulling

The life given us by nature is short, but the
memory of a well-spent life is eternal.

~CICERO

It is not doing the thing we like to do, but liking the
thing we have to do that makes life blessed.

~GOETHE

*A*cupuncture, aromatherapy, and pressure point massage: these are all natural Eastern-based healing modalities that you may have not only heard about but perhaps even have had some experience with these therapies. These, as well as many other ancient practices, have become more mainstream in Western society in recent years, mostly because, as you're most likely well aware, Americans are looking for alternatives to the doctors beholden to big pharma and their endless cycle of prescription meds, which often come with side effects as detrimental as the original malady. Not only that, but the ubiquity of information, accessible thanks to the internet, is helping to empower us to take our health into our own hands, enabling these ancient practices to finally make their long overdue comebacks.

Yet for all of our savvy these days, there are still many other ancient practices with which we may not yet be familiar. One of those is likely oil pulling. That's right, oil pulling. Although this may conjure up an image of cowboy hats and Dallas-style ranches, that locale couldn't be further from where this practice originated. Oil pulling is from the Ayurvedic tradition, the holistic medical practice, which began between 3,000 and 5,000 years ago in India and which has recently become popular here in the West with those of us seeking more natural remedies for serious diseases and illnesses, as well as for prevention. A quick Google search of oil pulling will yield hundreds of articles, yet somehow it has managed to stay under the radar in comparison to things like acupuncture, homeopathy, and others of the same ilk.

This is the practice you didn't know you were missing, but soon will wonder how you ever lived without it. For the initiated and uninitiated, here is a guide on what you need to know to get started with this at once ancient and trending practice.

Before we get into this topic, you might be interested in the webinar I presented entitled *ORAL CARE: Healthy Mouth – Healthy Body* (hosted by Hallelujah Diet), which I posted on my website. Simply put the words "Oral Care" in the search bar, and you'll find this informative, enlightening, and eye-opening presentation.

Here's a brief description of the webinar: Vibrant health really starts in the mouth! How you care for your teeth, gums, and tongue has a direct impact on your overall health. While a beautiful smile and fresh breath are often our main pursuits, this webinar extends our focus to include the gums, plaque, and more. Topics I discuss include how to keep your mouth healthy and pain-free; cavities; fillings, crowns and implants; oral irrigation; toothpaste and mouthwash; halitosis; how periodontal disease can be passed through kissing; teeth grinding; reasons to avoid sugar; jaw pain; nutritional supplements for strong choppers; motives for whitening and straightening teeth; and much more! You'll be inspired and motivated by what you learn and will be empowered to start taking better care of your oral hygiene. Get ready to be dazzled by the wealth of information!

Why Oil Pulling?

The list of benefits is quite remarkable when you consider how simple it is to oil pull. Among other advantages, oil pulling supports migraine headache relief; helps to balance hormones; aids in reduction of eczema; helps with gastroenteritis; promotes normal sleep patterns; relieves bad breath; supports body detoxification; reduces joint swelling; strengthens the teeth and jaws, prevents dry lips, throat and mouth; reduces bleeding gums; and more.

The following is a brief overview of oral care, heart health, and other possible benefits.

Oral Care

Anecdotal evidence about oil pulling's oral health care benefits is abundant and it's been used not just by practitioners of Ayurveda, but it's also been, you may be surprised to learn, used as a folk remedy here in America for a while now as well. In fact, I learned to do this as a teenager (and have been oil pulling for decades)—and from where would you guess I learned it? Well, it was my grandmother (Fritzie), not exactly someone who was otherwise an iconoclast against Western medicine, although she was into holistic health and raw foods. But Fritzie swore by it, and although I didn't see the point at the time, I now understand what a powerful practice it is. In fact, Fritzie lived to be quite a ripe old age. And unlike her peers, she never suffered major tooth decay, had no need for dentures and, in fact, had a beautiful smile up until her final years.

And now finally, recent scientific research has been provided to confirm what Fritzie, so many others, and I already knew. Studies prove that oil pulling not only destroys plaque, but also eliminates plaque-induced gingivitis and improves breath while functioning as nature's mouthwash. By absorbing the bacteria, the oil is able to neutralize and eliminate it by pulling it from deep dental crevices and gum tissue. And because it is a more concentrated and time-consuming process (don't worry, it's only slightly more time consuming, as you will learn soon) than brushing and cleansing with mouthwash, it makes sense that you're going to harvest and eliminate more of the bad bacteria and microorganisms than the conventional oral care regimen. Moreover, dentists are beginning to recognize the benefits of oil pulling and are even beginning to recommend it to patients, decidedly moving it out of the "alternative" health category and into the mainstream.

Heart Health

The link between heart health and oral care is quite well established. People with healthier mouths suffer from less heart disease and other coronary issues. So adding oil pulling to your daily routine is certainly going to up your oral care game, but it's also very likely going to protect your heart from dangerous bacteria as well.

Dentists and heart doctors have been exhorting heart patients for years now to become more cognizant of oral health in order to protect their hearts from bacteria. It makes since that if you kill bacteria in the mouth, you'll prevent it from moving to other parts of the body. And this is exactly the philosophy behind the idea that we need to take care of our oral hygiene in order to protect our hearts.

Researchers have proven that people with periodontal disease are twice as likely to have heart disease. Bacteria in the mouth can travel to the bloodstream, which obviously can affect your heart. In the fatty deposits that clog arteries (the condition known as atherosclerosis), doctors have found oral bacteria. This is remarkable and proof that oral bacteria seeping into the bloodstream makes its way to the heart. Although it's not the same kind, the fat buildup in the arteries where these oral bacteria sometimes end up, causing atherosclerosis, is often referred to as plaque. Perhaps conflating the two types of plaque in your mind though isn't such a bad thing since there is likely a link. By avoiding oral plaque buildup, you are probably also avoiding the cardiovascular variety as well. Furthermore, endocarditis, an infection in the heart, is caused directly by bacteria that often make their way into the bloodstream via the mouth.

Hopefully you've avoided heart issues thus far, but all of us, whether we're under the care of a cardiologist or not, can benefit from oil pulling's ability to kill oral bacteria. As we age, we become more prone to heart disease and its implications. Why not invest a little extra effort caring for this vital organ?

Other Health Benefits

They say, "The eyes are the window to the soul." Well although not as often heard, I'd like to add that "the mouth is the mirror of the body." In other words, oral health often reflects the body's general health conditions since this is where bacteria and other microorganisms enter our systems. If we don't neutralize these bacteria, they enter our system and the bloodstream, potentially wreaking havoc on our organs and bodily functions. This is the philosophy motivating many an oil-puller these days. And although only the claims regarding oral and heart health are as yet scientifically substantiated, it is very likely that the science affirming the practice's other benefits is on the horizon.

As we continue to claim our personal health power to improve our lives by taking our health care into our own hands through our diets and other daily habits, oil pulling is yet another tool to add to that powerful arsenal.

How and When to Enjoy Oil Pulling

So before we get into the nitty-gritty about what oil pulling can do for you, I'm going to explain *how* to do oil pulling so you can see how easy it is—and perhaps even go put some in your mouth right now and do it as you read the rest of this chapter. Why not? By the time you finish reading, you'll be on the road to better health and have a cleaner mouth (and perhaps system). And you likely have everything you need to do it already in your kitchen. That's the beauty of this simple yet transformative practice!

How to Oil Pull

Although the literature recommends using coconut oil (more on that to follow), you can also use sesame, sunflower, or olive oil. Simply place one tablespoon in your mouth. If you feel like a tablespoon is too much to hold in your mouth without swallowing, then start with a half. After some practice, you'll find it easier to hold it in your mouth without the danger of swallowing any. The reason to be careful is because you'll be swishing around the toxins that the oil is pulling out, so you obviously don't want to accidentally ingest them.

And although it's called oil pulling, it could alternatively be called oil swishing since that's what you're primarily doing. The pulling refers to the way you're supposed to pull it through your teeth. Mostly, you'll be swishing it around your tongue and over your gums, but remember to try to also pull it through your teeth. Take care not to do it too vigorously though because you'll want to prevent your jaw from getting tired (yes, this can happen) thus potentially causing you to give up early. Although keep in mind that exercising the ligaments and tendons around the jawline could strengthen your jaw and even save you money on cosmetic surgery! Seriously though, unless you want it to be, this doesn't have to be an athletic experience for your mandible. Gentle swishing is best to prevent fatigue. Twenty minutes is the ideal duration and the recommended time, which should yield the best results. However, you may need to work up to this. If five minutes feels like all you can handle, don't despair. You've certainly achieved some results. The next day try to do it a minute longer and continue like this until you get up to 20 minutes. Don't give up on the practice though if you never reach 20 minutes because benefits will still be yours as long as you do it for as few as 5 minutes a day (although, of course, 20 is optimal).

When to Oil Pull

Personally, I like to do it first thing in the morning while I'm getting my breakfast ready because that's when the most unfriendly and risky bacteria are teeming in our mouths. Before I do anything—drink water or even brush my teeth, I oil pull. Then when I'm done, I have my delicious, healthy breakfast as a reward as well as the exhilarating sense that I've accomplished something important, all before 7 a.m. A friend of mine who also does it in the morning claims that it's an excuse to not have to engage with the kids and hubby right away while she uses the time to get her bearings and wake up. She tells me that she cherishes the morning quiet time before she has to begin cajoling and prodding everyone to get on task. And she jokes that it's her jaw's morning training routine before she begins raising her voice at everyone.

Although I oil pull in the morning and that's what many practitioners recommend, especially because one of its supposed benefits is enhanced energy, it's not, however, at all necessary that you do it then. If the pre-breakfast morning time slot doesn't fit into your routine, no problem. The important thing is that you do it when it works for you. Since you want to focus on endurance and getting up to 20 minutes eventually, the trick is to find an activity that you can engage in while swishing that will keep you distracted—and, for many, this time is not upon waking up. Whatever time of day works for you, do it then, because, unfortunately, the bacteria are teeming all day. Cooking, watching television, gardening, knitting, even taking a showing, whatever your thing is, do it during an activity that you enjoy in order to keep yourself distracted, so you're not concentrating on every swish and pull, which can, of course, be tedious if your mind is not otherwise engaged. Personally, I've heard that the most compelling way to pass the time is by reading articles on the Susan Smith Jones website. People report walking away feeling healthier and smarter! 🙂

Finally, when it's time to spit out the oil, choose the trash can over the sink because when you begin to do this regularly, the oil in the sink could build up and cause a clog. Then, rinse your mouth with water before ingesting anything else in order to eliminate any remaining toxins. I always use warm water to which I've added a sprinkle of sea salt for rinsing my mouth about three times after oil pulling. And that's it. You just did your body a favor, the rewards for which are many. You should be feeling and seeing the benefits in no time.

Oil Types

Although all of the above mentioned oils—sesame, olive, sunflower, and coconut oil—have many of the same properties, which makes them all great candidates for your new habit, coconut oil is the one most recommended for one good reason: lauric acid. Lauric acid, one of the fatty acids found only in coconut oil, is an antimicrobial. What is an antimicrobial? Well, remember that one bacterium you're already acquainted with by name—*Streptococcus mutans*? Well guess what lauric acid's favorite activity is? That's right. It loves to kill all bacteria and fungi, and is especially good at eliminating the most virulent one, the streptococcus variety. Therefore, coconut oil is the mostly highly recommended of the oils. This bonus factor gives it heavy weight status amongst the other oils. I use raw, organic coconut oil exclusively for my oil pulling.

And since I suggest you swish for the full 20 minutes, you're more likely to accomplish this successfully with coconut oil since it definitely tastes the best. It always makes me feel a little like I'm at the beach because the taste of coconut oil reminds me of coconut trees in a tropical setting. Just always make sure that you choose an organic, raw, and non-GMO brand.

How Often Should You Swish?

So you've finished this chapter, and maybe your inaugural swishing session, and now you're wondering how often you need to do this. Most professionals I speak to about this recommend doing it at least a few times a week. I recommend doing it every day for the first month so that you can really see some tangible results and, thus, feel motivated to keep doing it into the future. After that first month, consider that you may only need to do it 3 to 5 times a week to maintain the benefits. Many people notice results within the first few days for one or more of the above-discussed oral benefits. How long you have to wait often has to do with the state of your current oral health. If your oral health is compromised or your oral health regimen has been lacking, you may need to have a bit more patience before seeing results.

Let's Review

❖ Place a half to a full tablespoon of coconut, sesame, sunflower, or olive oil in your mouth.

- Allow it to liquefy and then swish gently. Try to pull it through your teeth and around on your tongue and gums.

- Do this for no less than 5 minutes and up to 20. Remember, you want to avoid a tired jaw so be gentle. And avoid swallowing!

- When finished, spit the oil into the trash.

- Rinse your mouth with water when you're done. Don't drink or eat anything until you've rinsed away the remaining toxins.

- Brush your teeth. And don't forget to smile.

A Note about the Ayurvedic Method

Although oil pulling is an Ayurvedic practice no matter how you do it, the purist in you may desire to do it in the traditional fashion, which is slightly different from what I've outlined. Although many people I know who are steeped in Ayurvedic tradition prefer to practice it in the more modern way (the one I just described), I'll briefly review, for you traditionalists, the ancient method in case you feel inclined to practice in the same way as our incredible ancestors who invented this practice for us did!

OIL PULLING VS. MOUTHWASH

So you may be wondering—why not just use mouthwash and gargle and swish for a fraction of the time that oil pulling necessitates? Well, one very important reason is that mouthwash may be too good at killing bacteria. What I mean by that is that it kills *all* the bacteria—even the good kind. That may sound like an oxymoron—good bacteria. But, yes, similar to the gut, we need certain bacteria to maintain a healthy mouth. Mouthwash usage has even been linked to the development of health issues as serious as diabetes. Also, it's argued that mouthwash can stain teeth. Therefore, many dental professionals knowledgeable about oil pulling benefits would prefer that you oil pull than use mouthwash for those three important reasons.

Within the ancient tradition, there were two techniques called gandusa and kavala. In the gandusa method, one simply holds the oil in the mouth without swishing for 3 to 5 minutes before spitting it out and repeating the process. In kavala, you briefly hold the oil in the mouth before swishing it around for just a few minutes, then spit it out and repeat the process several more times.

More on Oral Health Benefits

A mouth full of bacteria and microorganisms can lead to many oral health implications. Swishing oil pulls these suckers out in a way that brushing and flossing alone can't. It's important to remember, however, that oil pulling should not be used as a substitute for brushing and flossing, which you should continue doing at least twice daily. Oil pulling is meant to complement your already thorough oral care practice. That is if you also want to soon be complimented on your beautiful pearly whites!

Gingivitis

Studies indicate that plaque-induced gingivitis is improved by oil pulling. It took just over a week in one study for participants using sesame oil to notice the reduction to both the plaque and gingivitis. Another study with coconut oil yielded similar results. Both studies revealed signs of improvement within the first 10 days. And in both monthlong studies, the results became even more dramatic as the study continued. It therefore doesn't take a logician to realize that plaque and plaque-related gingivitis are within your power to prevent if you regularly pull oil.

Tooth Decay

For many people, even those of us who romanticize certain historical eras, the offer to travel back in time would be one we might decline because we all know that those people had never heard of a toothbrush, had foul-smelling breath, and had mouths full of rotting teeth and bleeding gums? Right? Not so fast. What many people don't know is that the Romans are reported to have had perfect teeth, better even than ours! And they're not the only ones. Many other ancient cultures had no instances of tooth decay either and this is true even now for many modern indigenous people. There is a common belief that technology and modernity has led to improvements in just about every aspect of life compared to the past. However, although we may be able to extend our lives, we suffer many new ailments that were previously unknown (and are still unknown in other lands) and tooth decay is one of those afflictions.

So why do we take for granted that tooth decay is an inevitability? Because we try to rationalize that sugar, starch, and dairy are necessary, desirable even, aspects of our diets. The truth though is that they actually are avoidable and not inevitable components of the modern diet. And they are indeed the root causes of many of our modern ailments, including tooth decay.

The pernicious bacteria left behind on the teeth after ingesting these foods are what lead to tooth decay if not removed, as you will learn about from my oral care webinar mentioned earlier. So if you're not ready to completely transform your diet, then at least consider oil pulling. Although the scientific proof is still lacking, and we know that oil pulling will not reverse tooth decay, if it significantly reduces the bacteria enough to improve plaque and plaque-induced gingivitis, we can certainly assume that we are creating a generally healthier environment in our mouths. And potentially preventing tooth decay!

Halitosis

It's intuitive that if you kill millions of microbes in your mouth, you'll be improving your breath. Oral bacteria cause bad breath; therefore, eliminating them can improve your breath. My own interviews and conversations with people seem to bear this out. One friend even reported an improvement in her marriage. Apparently, the intimacy in her relationship had suffered due to her husband's repugnant-smelling breath. They'd tried everything and were prepared to visit their doctor when I recommended oil pulling. They were astonished at the immediate difference. Lo and behold, their love life was back on track and they're very grateful to have discovered such an affordable treatment. If you suspect that you are guilty of bad breath, or someone has been kind (or mean) enough to inform you of it, try adding oil pulling to your oral care regimen and see for yourself.

Sensitivity

Tooth and gum sensitivity circumscribes many lives because it limits what we can eat. Oil pulling has been reported to relieve this pain by reducing tooth and gum sensitivity and to this one, I can personally attest. For a time, I avoided cold foods. I had sacrificed strawberries and other cut fruits, which require refrigeration because of the sharp pain they caused to both my teeth and gums. I am happy to say that oil pulling has revolutionized my way of eating. Since I began doing the practice again regularly many years ago after discontinuing for a few years because of extensive traveling, I've found that the pain is gone and I readily enjoy these fruits again. And although, my savvy health readers, I know you would never indulge in ice cream (wink wink), it's nice to know you can if you are so inclined—or at least enjoy frozen fruit dessert like banana "ice cream." (And, okay, in the interest of full disclosure, it may have happened a time or two that those strawberries happened to be topping a bowl of ice cream even though mine was the nondairy kind. We've all got to indulge sometimes.)

Other Health Benefits

Streptococcus mutans, the same bacteria associated with tooth decay and which is responsible for heart issues, is also considered a culprit in quite a few other health conditions such as meningitis, sinusitis, and pneumonia. Studies are still needed to link these bacteria to other ailments. But until then we have our common sense. Bacteria in the bloodstream becoming lodged in the body, whether it's in tissue or organs, is obviously undesirable and already known to lead to a variety of health problems. Why would we want it floating around in there, potentially causing other issues? So although the following claims are as yet unverified by any scientific data, I'd like to briefly mention what some of the claims are that many people swear by.

Now that we understand how strongly bacteria is linked to disease, it's not hard to imagine that it is capable of at least throwing other things in the body out of whack—like hormones. Because oil pulling is detoxifying, hormone regulation is claimed by many as a benefit. Without bacteria in the mix, hormones can carry on unadulterated by foreign bodies. This is the same basis for claims about skin and skin clarity. Whether using it to get fresh, glowing, youthful skin or to clear up rashes, many users agree that they see improvements in skin quality after practicing oil pulling regularly. Other claims include relief from headaches, increased energy, and even weight loss.

Do your own investigation into the claims if you like. You may as well be conscious of them and see what else you notice since you're going to be oil pulling anyway because of the unequivocal oral benefits. One friend of mine who had a severe case of Lyme disease practiced oil pulling as part of her Ayurvedic regimen. She doesn't know what led to her improved health (she's been Lyme-free for several years now), but one can't discount that oil pulling may have been a factor.

Final Thoughts

It's not just the health of our mouths that are important; there's the aesthetic component as well. Our smiles are one of the first things people notice about us and are central to the impression we make. Our feelings about our teeth, too, can lead to confidence or, unfortunately, deflate it. Our teeth are a part of our bodies that many people attend to more than once a day. Most of us shower once a day, but brush our teeth twice or more. That's because of the traffic, so to speak, going on in there. And unlike other parts of our bodies, we notice it more when our mouths don't feel clean. Adding oil pulling to your regimen then makes a lot of sense. And, of course, we all want to avoid frequent dentist visits and painful oral surgery. As a holistic health care expert, this is one of the best health care practices I am aware of that we can easily and affordably do for ourselves at home. I can't wait for you to start seeing results for yourself.

To read my entire chapter on "ORAL CARE: Healthy Mouth – Healthy Body," please refer to my book *Body Temple Vitality*.

Blessed are the pure in heart, for they shall see God.
~MATTHEW 5:8

Taking the first footstep with a good thought, the second with a good word, and the third with a good deed, I entered Paradise.

~ZOROASTER

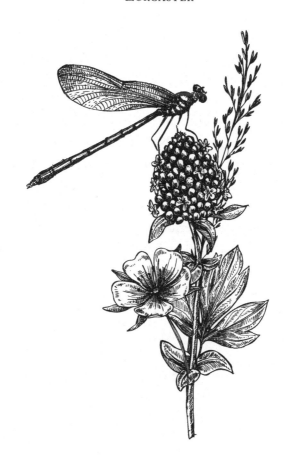

Humor Time, Part 1

*E*verybody loves to laugh. In fact, did you know that laughter is very good for you? It was Norman Cousins who said, "Laughter is a form of internal jogging." Humor and laughter have both been found to be important components of healing. It's been reported that laughter aids digestion, stimulates the heart, strengthens muscles, activates the brain's creative function, and keeps you alert. Laughter also helps you to keep things in better perspective. So make up your mind to laugh and to be happy. When you laugh at yourself, you take yourself far less seriously. "Angels fly because they take themselves lightly," says an old Scottish proverb. Isn't that wonderful?

I simply love to laugh and am known to be a practical joker! My mother, June, called laughter "the body's elixir" or natural rejuvenator. It is an essential ingredient to daily living and something I use to fuel my spirituality. Because of my positive, easygoing, "lighten up" approach to life, I have acquired the nickname "Sunny" because I am often reminding others to not take life so seriously.

So here is a funny story that might bring you a good laugh, too. Enjoy!

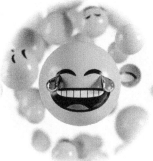

At the Gym for Christmas this Year

At the gym for Christmas this year, my wife purchased me a week of private lessons at the local health club. Though still in great shape from when I was on the varsity chess team in high school, I decided it was a good idea to go ahead and try it. I called and made reservations with someone named Tanya, who said she is a 26-year-old aerobics instructor and athletic clothing model. My wife seemed very pleased with how enthusiastic I was to get started.

Day 1: *They suggest I keep this "exercise diary" to chart my progress this week. Started the morning at 6:00 am. Tough to get up, but worth it when I arrived at the health club and Tanya was waiting for me. She's something of a goddess, with blond hair and a dazzling white smile. She showed me the machines and took my pulse after five minutes on the treadmill. She seemed a little alarmed that it was so high, but I think just standing next to her in that outfit of hers added about ten points. Enjoyed watching the aerobics class. Tanya was very encouraging as I did my sit ups, though my gut was already aching a little from holding it in the whole time I was talking to her. This is going to be great.*

Day 2: *Took a whole pot of coffee to get me out the door, but I made it. Tanya had me lie on my back and push this heavy iron bar up into the air. Then she put weights on it, for heaven's sake! Legs were a little wobbly on the treadmill, but I made it the full mile. Her smile made it all worth it. Muscles feel great.*

Day 3: *The only way I can brush my teeth is by laying the toothbrush on the counter and moving my mouth back and forth over it. I am sure that I have developed a hernia in both pectorals. Driving was okay as long as I didn't try to steer. I parked on top of a Volkswagen. Tanya was a little impatient with me and said my screaming was bothering the other club members. The treadmill hurt my chest so I did the stair monster. Why would anyone invent a machine to simulate an activity rendered obsolete by the invention of elevators? Tanya told me regular exercise would make me live longer. I can't imagine anything worse.*

Day 4: *Tanya was waiting for me with her vampire teeth in a full snarl. I can't help it if I was half an hour late; it took me that long just to tie my shoes. She wanted me to lift dumbbells. Not a chance, Tanya. The word "dumb" must be in there for a reason. I hid in the men's room until she sent Lars looking for me. As punishment she made me try the rowing machine. It sank.*

Day 5: *I hate Tanya more than any human being has ever hated any other human being in the history of the world. If there were any part of my body not in extreme pain I would hit her with it. She thought it would be a good idea to work on my triceps. Well, I have news for you, Tanya, I don't have triceps. And if you don't want dents in the floor don't hand me any barbells. I refuse to accept responsibility for the damage—you went to sadist school and you are to blame. The treadmill flung me back into a science teacher, which hurt like crazy. Why couldn't it have been someone softer, like a music teacher, or social studies?*

Day 6: *Got Tanya's message on my answering machine, wondering where I am. I lacked the strength to use the TV remote so I watched eleven straight hours of the weather channel.*

Day 7: *Well, that's the week. Thank goodness that's over. Maybe next time my wife will give me something a little more fun, like free teeth-drilling at the dentist's office.*

AFFIRMATION TO BRIGHTEN UP YOUR DAY

Repeat this affirmation three times silently or out loud whenever you start taking yourself and life too seriously:

I am laughing my way to a happy, gleeful day.
Laughter is the elixir for my soul. I look for the good in
others and bring humor to every circumstance. With
joy and lightheartedness, I celebrate this day.

Part 3

Make Balance,
Peace & Prosperity
Your Daily Companions

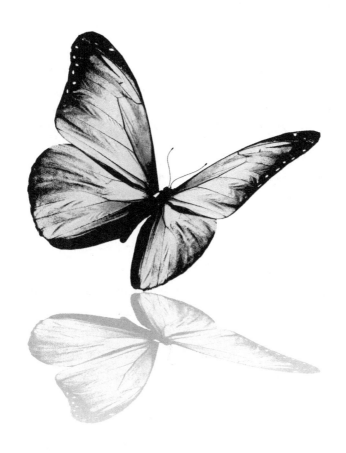

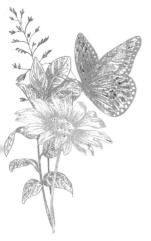

Chapter 7

Meditating through the Ages & World

Instead of concentrating on your problems and getting discouraged, focus on God and meditate on His promises for you. You may have fallen down, but you don't have to stay down. God is ready, willing, and able to pick you up.

~JOYCE MEYER

At the center of the Universe is a loving heart that continues to beat and that wants the best for every person. Anything that we can do to help foster the intellect and spirit and emotional growth of our fellow human beings, that is our job. Those of us who have this particular vision must continue against all odds. Life is for service.

~FRED ROGERS

About 20 years ago, I was on a flight to give talks at three Christian churches, a Fortune 500 company, and two women's groups. It just so happened that I was carrying with me a magazine in which there was an interview I had given and which featured me on the cover. I was reading the interview I had given for the first time when a seemingly kind and pleasant gentleman sat down next to me and introduced himself. When he glanced over at the magazine I was reading, he seemed delighted to see that I was the subject of the interview and exclaimed, "How lucky I am to be sitting next to a celebrity." I explained that I was not a celebrity but told him that I was just reading the interview

I had given three months prior in a three-hour sit-down and photoshoot.

When he asked if he could read it after I finished, I agreed since I was quite proud of the comprehensive and positive content of the interview. One of the questions the interviewer had asked of me was about how I stayed connected and engaged when life got stressful. I discussed the importance of sleep and exercise as well as meditation. Specifically I said, "It's a simple, cost-free, and effective way to quiet my mind by closing my eyes and breathing slowly and deeply. Focusing on my breath is an easy way to shut out the chaos of the world for a few moments of joyful quiet stillness. And for me, I turn within to connect with the peace and love of God that is a guiding light in my life." Then I mentioned a couple more things about how meditation has helped me stay strong, collected, and peaceful over the decades and how I had taught workshops worldwide on this subject and even made house calls to teach families and individuals how to meditate.

When my fellow passenger finished reading, he suddenly called to the flight attendant to ask for a new seat. I was astonished, to say the least, but kept very quiet. When the flight attendant asked him what the issue was he replied, "The issue is that this lady sitting next to me is evil and related to the devil because she meditates and it's against my religion to associate with or talk to any crazy person who practices devil worship."

Well needless to say, I was dumbfounded. As a health practitioner, writer, and speaker, my focus has never been anything but promoting well-being and positivity; his words were ones I'd never heard ascribed to me and certainly never anticipated ever hearing. If the gentleman had remained next to me, I would have taken the opportunity to explain to him that meditation is scientifically proven to alleviate the symptoms of many physical and mental issues and even to slow down the aging process. We could have also discussed the fact that meditation has not historically been at odds with Christianity, and in fact, there are specific philosophies about and ways to practice Christian meditation. But, unfortunately, he had been indoctrinated to believe that meditation is a heretical act.

But that's not the end of the story. After he moved his seat, most of the people sitting around me, including three of the flight attendants, who heard his clamorous judgments of me took turns sitting in his empty seat to ask me their personal questions about meditation. Each person wanted my guidance on how they could meditate and how they could teach it to their loved ones, children, colleagues, and more. It was very gratifying. Fortunately, it was a long flight to NYC, so I had time to speak with many other passengers about meditation, living peacefully, and creating high-level wellness.

Although this occurred 20 years ago, the experience has stayed with me and is one I often recall with some sadness because I believe that this man as well as many others are really missing out on a transformative experience—and one that really could have offered him a way to enrich his faith. So I've finally decided that, although it's overdue, it's time to offer some insight about the relationship between meditation and the world's most practiced religions, it's ancient history as well as its many benefits.

So without further ado . . .

A History of Meditation

Before I go into the history of meditation, perhaps you may be keen on knowing when I first learned about it and started practicing meditation. When I was a teenager, my grandmother, Fritzie, taught me about the importance of meditation and how to meditate simply and easily and incorporate it into my lifestyle. She taught me that the word "yoga" means "union" and that it refers to a union with God and a union of the body, mind, and spirit. Learning the importance of breathing deeply, especially when life gets overwhelming and filled with stress, was another one of her many teachings in my life for which I am so grateful. (To learn more about my life-changing and life-enriching relationship with my grandmother and also how she taught me about kitchen gardening—how to grow culinary herbs and sprouts like alfalfa, broccoli, lentil, garbanzo, etc.—please refer to my book *Kitchen Gardening*.)

We hear a lot about meditation these days. Despite the fact that it's been around for thousands of years, it's not been practiced widely in the Western world except for in small religious and spiritual pockets. But as modern life continues to speed up, commanding more commitments while offering less time for self, meditation has become a popular palliative to relieve stress. The resurgence of yoga in the nineties is likely the way more Americans began to become familiar with meditation, which is fundamentally a moving meditation. But lately, meditation is commonly being practiced independently of yoga. In fact, it is quite ubiquitous in America today, and in any metropolitan city you can find a handful of meditation studios as well as meetup and other community groups offering meditation classes and sessions. And we may laugh at the irony, but there are literally hundreds of phone apps devoted just to meditation. As meditation begins to become more acceptable, even to many Christians who once condemned it as "evil," and begins to be adopted by corporate America and even the government who offer quiet rooms for meditation, it's pretty clear that meditation is not a fad that's going away anytime soon.

So as it becomes more a part of everyday life, people have begun to wonder about its origins and how it has evolved over the years. You might be surprised to learn that it's thought that hunter-gatherers even practiced some form of meditation. The earliest recordings of meditation are not even written but in hieroglyph form. Earlier meditators who were nonverbal may have been practicing a form of meditation as they slipped into an altered consciousness through staring at the fire. But theorists believe this iteration of our ancestors had no need for meditation in the way we employ it now or even the way we did 5,000 years ago because essentially, meditation is an exercise in quieting the noise of the mind—which we wouldn't have if we didn't have that pesky thing called language.

So how does a practice that was discovered/invented by primitive humans still appeal to modern humans who don't recognize much of themselves in these early ancestors. In a world filled with VR, CGI, and AI (virtual reality, computer generated images, and artificial intelligence), we've obviously evolved right? Well, our technology may have, but we are still unchanged in most aspects. And, ironically, all that technology is compelling a need to return to simplicity and for mental calm. Lions trying to kill you may not be the stressor triggering that need anymore, but there is still a need. Meditation has evolved over the years to fit the varying needs of the societies and eras it's been practiced in. And it's a fascinating evolution.

Meditation—From Caves to the Pentagon: Let's Connect Those Dots!

The word *meditation* stems from *meditatum*, a Latin term that means "to ponder." Through my personal practice of daily meditation for decades and also from working with countless other people worldwide to support them in cultivating the presence of God through meditation, I am keenly aware how it helps us to find a better connection with our body in the everyday moments that we often let pass us by, and create stronger awareness for how our mental perspective and emotions influence our behavior. It was Michel de Montaigne, a French philosopher, who once said, "The greatest thing in the world is to know how to belong to oneself." Living in such a fast-paced world, often in one tizzy after another with so many demands on our minds and our time, it truly takes a conscious commitment and effort to set aside a few moments to ourselves to explore our inner worlds and be at peace in our own company. This health-enhancing and life-enriching process of meditation has been part of the history of the world and every culture in one form or another. Let's explore some of the historical particulars of this healing discipline.

Meditation: The Very Early Years

Although it's only a theory, some scientists subscribe to the idea that meditation was the thing that separated us from our Neanderthal relatives. Once they had fire, these prehistoric humans had a reason to come together at night and form a community. Focused attention on the fire led to a kind of meditation (we all know about the hypnotic power of watching a fire). Since meditation is actually associated with improved memory, researchers' theory stipulates that the focused attention on fire led to the development of stronger memories and is what eventually began separating us modern humans from our Neanderthal ancestors about 200,000 years ago. Psychologist and author of the book *Supernatural Selection*, Matt J. Rossano, was the first to propose this theory. He argues that rituals then developed from this communal activity and the brain continued to develop its cognitive functions over subsequent millennia. Hence, he believes that religion, and to go back further, meditation, are what led to the cognitive development necessary for evolution and which separated us from our more primitive ancestors.

Original Practitioners

More recently, if you can call 7,000 years ago recently, practitioners of meditation documented the experience not in writing but in wall paintings. These depict figures in cross-legged seated positions with half-closed eyes, the same posture many use now for meditation. The first documented records, however, of meditation come from the Vedas, the first Hindu scriptures written in the Indian subcontinent between 1,500 and 1,000 BC. This is the reason we associate the East with meditation because it is indeed where it first formally began; even the earlier wall paintings were in this region. It's believed that between the time of the pictorial renderings of meditation found in caves and the written strictures found in the Vedas, the tradition was passed on orally. Scholars confirm that in the time before written texts like the Vedas, humans had been engaging in various forms of meditative activities such as chanting, rhythmic drumming, and other activities that can induce a trance-like state.

Getting back to the Vedas, the texts themselves are the documentation of ancient sages' revelations that they actually derived from deep meditation. They are part of a collection of other scripture that influenced the still-thriving religion of Hinduism. That ancient form of meditation has seen a resurgence since the 1960s when Maharishi Mahesh Yogi rebranded it for the west as Transcendental Meditation.

Nowadays, Transcendental Meditation, or TM as it is popularly known, is synonymous with Vedic meditation, and the terms are used interchangeably. In this form of meditation, a mantra is repeated over and over again in the mind. The emphasis is not on eliminating thoughts since this tradition believes that the attempt to completely clear the mind takes a certain amount of force and discipline, which in most cases, undermines attempts at the cessation of thought. This tradition instead emphasizes the repetition of the mantra as a way to quiet the thoughts. Deepak Chopra describes it this way:

As you repeat the mantra, it creates a mental vibration that allows the mind to experience deeper levels of awareness. As you meditate, the mantra becomes increasingly abstract and indistinct, until you're finally led into the field of pure consciousness from which the vibration arose. Repetition of the mantra helps you disconnect from the thoughts filling your mind so that perhaps you may slip into the gap between thoughts.

Buddhism

For many, when they think of Buddhism, meditation is the first thing that comes to mind, likely because the icons and statues of Buddha almost exclusively depict him in meditation. It's believed that the Buddha probably learned meditation from wandering Hindu aesthetes in the sixth century BC. The Buddha is known to have gained enlightenment through meditation. In fact, the eight-fold path of Buddhism is comprised of three basic divisions, one being meditation, which is considered essential for freedom from earthly suffering, the core ethos of Buddhism. It is important to note that the Buddhist tradition of meditation is distinguished from the Hindu tradition in that Buddhism does not believe there is one organizing principle in the universe such as a god. The emphasis therefore is not on finding union with God but rather on enlightenment, seeking truth, and tranquility through nonattachment. The popularity of the Buddha's teaching inspired many all across India and eventually spread to China and Japan where they developed their own traditions, meditation remaining at the heart.

Judaism

Interestingly, it is believed that the traditions from which Judaism arose in the fifth and sixth century BC practiced meditation and the burgeoning religion adopted it. An important aspect of Judaism is deep reflection on God, and meditation is often employed as a method for seeking the divine. The Old Testament actually uses the word "meditation" 23 times. However, its use is not always regarding the act of meditation that we think of in the Eastern sense but rather often used as a synonym for "reflect," as in "I meditate on your precepts and consider your ways," a phrase found in the Psalms.

There are, though, a variety of forms of meditation associated with Judaism, and the concept of mindfulness, which we normally associate with Buddhism, is also woven into the Torah. Although it is not necessarily widely practiced among Jews, many in the more deeply religious communities such as Orthodox and Hasidic regularly meditate using the various forms from the teachings. One such form is a meditation similar to Buddhist meditation, which focuses on the breath and eliminating thought. What distinguishes the two religions' approaches to meditation is that Jewish practitioners, every few cycles of breath, will remember the creator and sometimes mentally recite a line from the Torah. Additionally, students of Kabbalah, the mystical interpretation of the Bible, who are not always necessarily Jewish, also practice meditation.

Islam

The prophet Mohammed practiced meditation as a way to seek union with the divine. Meditation techniques mostly developed among Sufis, the Muslims who focused on the mystical aspects of Islam in the eleventh and twelfth centuries. The meditations they practiced, and still practice, focus, as Mohammed did, on union with God. And many also incorporate breathing techniques and mantras. However, this is controversial and many Muslims now debate whether they should be meditating at all because they see it as something too associated with Eastern religions. However, most scholars believe it to be an important aspect of the religion.

Christianity

The Islamic debate about meditation's role in the religion is not unlike the one in Christianity. Many people nowadays practice a very secular form of meditation. Since the nineties, meditation has become so much more widespread that most people don't even associate it with the New Age movement anymore and often use it for stress relief and for deeper connection to God. Yet, the practice still resembles Eastern traditions in its focusing on the breath, a mantra, and/or detachment. This is the problem that some Christian groups have with meditation. They believe that emptying the mind, oneness with God, and even trying to relieve stress are dangerous activities that take the focus off of Christ. They see modern problems like stress as really being borne of pride and a lack of reverence of Christ. If they just return to Christ, humbling themselves before Him, they will find peace. They believe that meditation is a hubristic subversion of God because of its focus on connecting to Him when they should be humbling themselves before Him.

Historically though, Christians have included meditation in their worship. Monastic life in the Middle Ages is where Lectio Divina developed. The concept's four steps—read, meditate, pray, and contemplate—are meant to create communion with God. Various religious figures and monks promoted it over the years through texts and practice, and it became an important aspect of Catholic life. In the nineteenth century it was being practiced by many Protestants as well.

But despite their suspicions about the types of meditation being practiced by many secular people nowadays, Christians do indeed practice meditation, just one centered on the word of God. Rather than emptying the mind or even attempting to find connection with God, the focus is on a word or verse from the Bible that is to be repeated in the mind while considering how one might apply the teaching to his or her own life. Some Christians are carefully on guard though against letting the repeated word lose its meaning so that it simply becomes a mantra that empties the mind of other thoughts or allows for the meditator to enter an altered state of mind.

And there are many Christians who do indeed actually practice more Eastern-based forms of meditation, as they don't necessarily see a conflict between the clearing of the mind and focusing on the breath or a mantra and their religious beliefs. There are even many Christians who do, in fact, find compatibility between not just Eastern meditation and Christianity but between Buddhism itself and the Christian religion and who don't necessarily find it anathema to their religion.

Wherever you stand in this debate, there is a meditation style that works for everyone's religious status. Whether you use it to feel the power of Christ in your life, to find union with God, to calm your mind and body, to connect more deeply with your inner Light, or even all of the above, the benefits are manifold.

What Science Says about Meditation

Scientific evidence for the benefits of meditation are plentiful and actually quite mind-blowing! Since meditation is a means to relax and calm the mind, you might guess that it is quite beneficial for mental issues such as depression and anxiety. But what you probably wouldn't guess is that is has been proven to offer benefits for a multitude of physical disorders. High blood pressure, ulcerative colitis, and irritable bowel syndrome are just a few of the physical ailments that studies have found meditation to be beneficial for. It also has been proven to ease symptoms of menopause. Furthermore, inflammation is said to be affected by meditation, and this is of great significance because inflammation is the underlying cause of the majority of diseases. Reducing inflammation is the one of the most important steps in boosting the immune system. We can easily infer, therefore, that meditation's medical benefits extend beyond what science has thus far been able to prove. And here's something that should appeal to most everyone: researchers have found proof that meditation can slow, and even, wait for it—reverse aging!

But getting back to the cognitive benefits, scientists have found evidence that meditation leads to the improvement of dozens of brain-related functions as well as promoting general emotional well-being. For example, studies have found that people who meditate regularly are better at processing information, controlling pain, and even sleep better and have better attention spans than those who don't. Researchers even found that meditation leads to improved social connections and that it actually generates kindness. I wish I had gotten the chance to communicate that to my fellow passenger, as that should allay the fear of those skeptics who believe that meditating is an invocation of evil.

Meditation's Modern Appeal & Application

In 2012, around 4% of Americans had some type of meditation practice. That number has increased at least 10% since then and is continuing to grow. And even kids are doing it. Around 5% add a little *omm* to their lives these days. As more parents discover the benefits of meditation for themselves, they're beginning to recognize that meditation has the potential to help with their kids' issues such as ADD, hyperactivity, behavioral issues, and just their general well-being.

Companies and corporations have also taken note and recognized the opportunity to improve their workers' overall well-being and thus enhance their job performances. Accordingly, many companies have introduced meditation programs to help their employees find more "zen" at work through wellness programs, meditation classes, or even just a quiet meditation room on the premises. Some such large-scale companies are Google, Nike, Apple, Yahoo, and HBO. By helping their workers deal with stress, these companies realize that they are not only creating happy workers but maximizing their productivity as well. Studies bear this out by revealing that employees with workplace meditation programs or rooms report less stress, increased focus, better ability to manage interoffice relationships, increased creativity, and even an overall better workplace culture. Rather than being a large expense for a company, which it may be initially, these programs ultimately save money by not only increasing employees' quality and quantity of output, but decrease worker burnout, and therefore, eliminate an excess of sick days.

Similarly, schools around the country are teaching meditation and implementing it to increase students' focus and improve their behavior. The practice in many schools also includes some yoga and stretching.

But it's the overall idea of mindfulness that administrators have identified as having a significant impact on students. Many schools are actually replacing detentions with meditation, offering kids a quiet place to reflect and to help them regulate their emotions, since this is one of the many benefits of meditation.

As we know, the lack of ability to control or understand emotions are often what lead troubled children to become troubled adults who find themselves continuing to experience antisocial behaviors, the kind that society sometimes punishes with a prison sentence. Like detention, the purely punitive approach to intolerable behavior offers little chance for rehabilitation. So prisons now have begun incorporating meditation programs for prisoners. These programs have been unequivocally successful. Not only does it does help prison guards more easily manage this notoriously unruly population, many studies have found a link between meditation and a reduction in violence and crime in general. Believe it or not, studies have found that prisoners who learn meditation while in prison experience much less recidivism. Better impulse control is the main reason cited by experts, since this is an inevitable outcome of meditation.

Finally, in one of the least expected locales on the planet, the Pentagon, generals, admirals, and high-ranking government officials are channeling meditation's benefits to better run the country and protect our national security. There are meditation rooms on the premises and there have even been conferences on the activity. If that doesn't sell you on the idea that meditation is actually a fairly mainstream activity nowadays, well then nothing will.

Meditation and You

So now that we've determined that meditation is not a heretical activity, but in fact, a deeply spiritual one for all religions and offers infinite possibilities for improved mental, physical, and emotional health for the majority of people, it's time to figure out the best way to incorporate meditation into your own life. As many types and approaches as there are to meditation, there are even more videos, books, internet sites, apps, etc. to help you get started. But then again, you may just not need to complicate the process. All you need is a quiet space, a comfortable place to sit, and your breath—and you can get started right away. You're already endowed with all of the equipment.

As we get older and wiser, many of us are making adjustments to our lives and adopting healthier habits. And this is one that I can guarantee you'll still be doing by year's end. It's free and easy and the many benefits are just waiting for you! Now's the time. I am excited for and support you on your new journey! And just in case you need one more excellent reason to welcome meditation in your lifestyle, this might do it: America's favorite medical doctor, Dr. Oz, encourages meditation for everyone to support a healthy immune system.

For detailed information on how to meditate easily, naturally and effortlessly, please refer to my audio program *Wired to Meditate* available at SusanSmithJones.com.

Dreams are the touchstones of our character.
~HENRY DAVID THOREAU

True beauty is not related to what color
your hair is or what color your eyes are.
True beauty is about who you are as a human
being, your principles, your moral compass.
~ELLEN DEGENERES

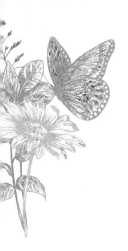

Chapter 8

Fostering a Soul-Satisfying Life with Meditation

Spending time with God is the key to our strength and success in all areas of life. Be sure that you never try to work God into your schedule, but always work your schedule around Him.

~JOYCE MEYER

To see the world in a grain of sand,
And heaven in a wild flower,
Hold infinity in the palm of your hand,
and eternity in an hour.

~WILLIAM BLAKE

$\mathcal{A}$s mentioned in the previous chapter, meditation is an ancient art that goes back long before recorded history. And here's a tad more history and science to help you lean more in the direction of meditation in your daily life.

Stone seals dating back to at least 5,000 BC have been found in the Indus Valley of India, showing people seated in various yoga postures. For all these millennia, meditation has survived as a vital science of living. This is not because meditation is esoteric or exotic or exclusively for monks and yogis, but because anybody can do it, and the benefits are perfectly clear to anybody who observes them.

Only during the past four decades, however, has scientific study focused on the clinical effects of meditation on health. The August 4,

2003, cover story of *Time* by Joel Stein was titled "The Science of Meditation" with the caption: "New Age mumbo jumbo? Not for millions of Americans who meditate for health and well-being." Scientists study it; doctors recommend it; millions of Americans and Britons—many of whom don't even own crystals—practice it daily. Why? Because meditation works! In fact, scientists have now developed tools sophisticated enough to see what goes on in your brain when you engage in a consistent meditation program.

In a nutshell: One study found that after training in meditation for eight weeks, subjects showed a pronounced change in brain-wave patterns, shifting from the beta waves of aroused, conscious thought to the alpha and theta waves that dominate the brain during period of deep relaxation. Sound intriguing? Read on.

Meditation is so thoroughly effective in reducing stress and tension, for example, that in 1984 the National Institutes of Health (NIH) recommended meditation over prescription drugs as the first treatment for mild hypertension. The late Dr. Hans Selye, a pioneering Canadian stress researcher, described two types of stress: negative stress and positive stress. The difference between the two depends upon whether or not we feel in control of the stress. Meditation, by making us more aware of our reactions to stress, can lead us toward an increased internal sense of control.

Health Benefits of Meditation

Dr. R. Keith Wallace at the University of California, Los Angeles, conducted the first research on the physiology of meditation. Studying Transcendental Meditation, Wallace found that during meditation the body arrives at a state of profound rest while the brain and mind become more alert, indicating a state of "restful alertness." Studies showed that after meditation, people exhibit faster reactions, greater creativity, and broader comprehension. Dr. Herbert Benson, formerly of the Mind-Body Medical Institute at Harvard University (MBMI), determined that meditation practice can bring about a healthy state of relaxation by causing a generalized reduction in physiological and biochemical stress indicators. Among the favorable indications are decreased heart rate, decreased respiration rate, decreased plasma cortisol (a stress hormone), decreased pulse rate, increased alpha waves (a brain wave associated with relaxation), and increased oxygen consumption.

Scientists are finding that meditation also helps keep us young and wrinkle-free. One study showed that people who had been meditating for more than five years were biologically 12 to 15 years younger than people who don't meditate. A comparison of the hospital records of 2,000 meditators and 2,000 non-meditators revealed that the meditators required only half as much medical care. They had 87 percent less heart disease, 55 percent fewer tumors, and 87 percent fewer nervous disorders.

JUST A FEW OF THE BENEFITS OF MEDITATION

❖ Faster reaction time

❖ Greater creativity

❖ Broader comprehension

❖ Lowered stress

❖ Decreased heart rate

❖ Decreased respiration rate

❖ Decreased cortisol

❖ Decreased pulse rate

❖ Increase in alpha waves in the brain (key to relaxation)

❖ Increased oxygen consumption

Another medical expert who advocates meditation is Dean Ornish, MD, a well-known physician and author of many books. In his path-paving book, *Dr. Dean Ornish's Program for Reversing Heart Disease*, there are easy-to-follow instructions for a calming routine that includes meditation, yoga, and progressive relaxation. So effective is his program that I sent my mother to attend one of his 7-day residential lifestyle retreats in Northern California; she returned with a new glow and commitment to healthy living.

Jon Kabat-Zinn, MD, at the University of Massachusetts Medical School, author of *Wherever You Go There You Are*, founded the

Stress Reduction Clinic in 1979 to help people suffering from chronic pain and chronic diseases such as cancer and heart disease, as well as stress-related disorders such as abdominal pain, chronic diarrhea, and ulcers. According to Dr. Kabat-Zinn, these conditions are often the most difficult to treat, and the patients have frequently tried other, more conventional forms of medicine without complete success.

Kabat-Zinn designed a stress-reduction program to test the value of using mindfulness meditation as an aid to patients in developing effective coping strategies for stress and to see whether meditation would have any effect on their various chronic medical conditions. His stress-reduction program patients had to make a commitment to practice on their own each day. As it turned out, the majority of people improved in a number of different ways:

❖ Virtually all patients, whatever their diagnoses, showed a dramatic reduction in physical symptoms over the eight-week period.

❖ Psychological problems—anxiety, depression, hostility—also dropped over the eight weeks. Follow-up studies four years after completion of the course showed that both physical and psychological improvements were consistent over time.

❖ Symptom reductions were greater than with other techniques such as drug intervention, indicating that the results were not coming from a placebo effect. Somehow the patients' inner resources for healing were being tapped.

❖ Patients' self-perceptions changed. They viewed themselves as healthier and better able to handle stressful situations without suffering destructive effects. They felt more in control of their lives, viewed life as a challenge rather than as a series of obstacles, and felt they were living more fully.

In general, Kabat-Zinn concludes that meditation is effective in decreasing pain, reducing the secretion of stress hormones including adrenaline and noradrenaline, decreasing the amount of excess stomach acid in people with gastrointestinal problems, lowering blood pressure, and increasing relaxation.

Managing Cancer with Meditation

Another study from the Tom Baker Cancer Centre in Calgary, Canada, has shown that meditation can substantially reduce levels of emotional distress and stress-related symptoms like headache, muscle tension, and stomach upset in patients undergoing chemotherapy.

As reported in *Psychosomatic Medicine*, researchers randomly assigned 90 cancer patients to one of two groups. The first group attended a meditation class once a week for seven weeks and was encouraged to meditate at least 30 minutes daily at home. The second group did not attend classes or receive instruction. Those who meditated experienced a major reduction in feelings of anger, depression, fatigue, and anxiety, and enjoyed a 31% drop in headaches, digestive problems, and racing heart.

Meditation and the Breath

Although there are many approaches to meditation, they can generally be grouped into two basic techniques: concentrative meditation and mindfulness meditation. Both are directed toward focusing the attention and strengthening the concentration, with the goal of quieting the mind to stillness.

Concentrative meditation focuses the attention on the breath, on an image, or on a sound (mantra) in order to slow the mind's activity and allow a greater awareness and clarity to emerge. To sit quietly and focus on your breath is the simplest form of concentrative meditation. This technique of meditation can be compared to the zoom lens of a camera that narrows its focus to a selected field.

Concentration is the ability to tell yourself to pay attention to something and then do exactly that! Our errant minds tend to drift. We have continuous mental conversations. Most people talk to themselves nearly every minute of the day. Through meditation we can limit, control, and finally eliminate this internal chitchat.

An effective way to control and master your mind is through breath awareness. The connection between the breath and one's state of mind is a basic principle of both yoga and meditation. Think back to a time when you were frightened, agitated, distracted, or anxious. Whether or not you noticed it then, your breath was probably shallow, rapid, and uneven, and you could probably duplicate those stressful emotions simply by breathing in a ragged, arrhythmic way. When the mind is focused and composed, the breath tends to be slow, deep, and regular. Working in reverse in just the same way, you can calm your mind by consciously taking slow, deep, and regular breaths. The continuous rhythm of inhalation and exhalation provides a natural focus for the mind, which facilitates meditation.

> Breath control is an amazing tool that allows you to alter your existing mental state.

Breath control is an amazing tool that allows you to alter your existing mental state. Inhale slowly and rhythmically through your nose, breathing quietly and deliberately. The incoming breath fills, in sequence, the abdomen, the ribcage, and the upper chest. After you draw a full, comfortable breath, hold it for a count of three, then let the air out slowly at the same rate and rhythm as the intake. The exhalation order is the exact reverse of the inhalation, in that the air leaves the upper chest, then the ribcage, and finally the abdomen. Allow the abdomen rather than the chest wall to power the breathing process, and try to breathe silently.

Breathe with concentration for a few minutes. Do it now. Settle into a comfortable posture and relax, but don't slump. Sit on a bench or chair with knees uncrossed and feet flat on the floor, or cross-legged on the floor on a cushion, folded towels, or a pillow. I sit on a chair sometimes, or on the floor on a quarter-moon-shaped pillow. The crossed-leg position, with buttocks slightly elevated, is great for smooth breathing and proper posture. Place your hands in one of two positions: the Zen mudra position, which is right hand palm up on the lap, left hand on top of right hand, also palm up, with the balls of the thumbs touching lightly. The alternate hand position is left hand on left thigh, right hand on right thigh, both with palms up, gently touching the thumb of each hand to the index finger. Doing nothing but monitoring your breathing, maintaining proper posture, and using one of the hand positions, you stay alert and focused. You are meditating. Notice as you do this that your mind becomes more tranquil and aware.

Mindfulness Meditation

The other type of meditation is mindfulness meditation. According to Dr. Joan Borysenko, author of *Inner Peace for Busy People*, mindfulness meditation involves opening your mind's attention to become aware of the continuously passing parade of sensations and feelings, images, thoughts, sounds, smells, and so forth without becoming involved in thinking about them or giving them our judgments. The meditator sits quietly and simply witnesses whatever goes through the mind, not reacting or becoming emotionally involved with thoughts, memories, worries, or images. This helps the meditator gain a calmer, clearer, and less reactive state of mind. Mindfulness meditation can be likened to a wide-angle lens—a broad, sweeping awareness that takes in the entire field of perception without concentrating on any one thing.

Mindfulness is an ancient Buddhist practice that has profound relevance for today, says Kabat-Zinn. Mindfulness has nothing to do with becoming a Buddhist, he points out, but is a way of "waking up and living in harmony with oneself and with the world." Living mindfully is paying complete attention to whatever we're doing, allowing the "mind to be full" of the experience. We are often more asleep than awake to the unique beauty and possibilities of each present moment as it unfolds. We're usually absorbed in anticipating the future—planning strategies to ward off things we don't want to happen and to force outcomes that we do want—or in remembering who did what to whom and why in the past. Such mental gymnastics can leave us exhausted, or at the very least nettled. Most of us spend very little time being aware of the present moment.

The opposite of mindfulness is mindlessness—doing things without thinking, without much feeling, automatically, and unconsciously like a robot. Although it is the tendency of our mind to go on automatic pilot, we can also call on our mind to help us awaken to each present moment and use it to advantage. We need to cultivate these moments of mindfulness because they are truly the only moments we have in which to live, grow, feel, love, learn, create, and heal. Coming out of automatic pilot and observing more deeply allows us to feel more connected to what's going on around us and to develop a greater understanding of the order of things. In mindfulness, we examine who we are, reevaluate our view of the world and our place in it, and learn how to appreciate the fullness of each moment we are alive.

When you practice mindfulness, you are in touch at all times with yourself and your surroundings, but just as a garden requires tending if you hope to grow flowers and not weeds, mindfulness requires regular cultivation. It doesn't happen all by itself. The beauty of it is that you carry this garden with you wherever you go, wherever you are, whenever you remember to explore it. It is outside of time as well as in it. Kabat-Zinn calls this mind cultivation "wakefulness meditation." You will find that the meditative disciplines, whether they involve mindfulness or concentrative techniques, bring calmness and stability into life.

Where to Meditate

It isn't necessary to travel to the Holy Land or the Himalayas to find a good meditation space. Dean Ornish began setting aside a space at home for his meditations when he was an undergraduate in college. "I was living in a one-bedroom apartment," he says, "and I didn't have a room I could use for that purpose. I didn't even have a corner of a room. But I had two closets. One I used for clothing; the other was for meditation." He recommends dedicating some space exclusively to prayer or meditation. Doing so enhances the meditation and makes not only that space but the home around it more sacred.

It's easy to create a personal sacred space. Ornish suggests, "You can put up a picture of a religious or holy person, or someone whose image evokes a sense of calmness or peace and love, or just set up a candle—whatever has the meaning for you of being sacred or inspiring."

A sacred place is where you find tranquility, where you will relish moments of rich solitude. "In your sacred space, things are working in terms of your dynamic and not anybody else's," explains Joseph Campbell. "Your sacred space is where you can find yourself again and again." And to this I would add that in your personal, sacred space, you always return to God.

For some uplifting and practical material on effective meditation and prayer, I recommend my audio programs *Wired to Meditate* and *Choose to Live Peacefully.*

How to Begin

I have been a disciplined meditator for the past 40 years, and for 30 years I've been a meditation counselor, conducting workshops and seminars in the U.S., U.K., and worldwide, as well as working one-on-one with individuals and families on simple ways to practice meditation to foster health, joy, and peace. So you see, I've benefited from decades of firsthand experience on the efficacy of meditation and how to incorporate it into busy lifestyles. You can learn about my experiences and how to meditate with ease and grace in my audio program *Wired to Meditate.* Here's a brief summary to get you started:

First, decide where you are going to meditate and create an altar for yourself. It can be decorated with uplifting books, pictures, or objects such as statues, candles, or flowers—anything that makes you feel serene—but keep it simple and clean. For more than 30 years I have set aside a corner of my bedroom as my place of meditation. On my altar (which is really an upside-down wicker basket) I have placed a natural cloth covering and some items that inspire me, including pictures of Jesus, the Bible, a candle, and some fresh flowers. I sit on the floor, as I said, on a pillow designed for meditation—but sometimes I will also opt to sit in a chair, too. Make sure the seat of the chair is parallel to the floor and that your spine is straight. In other words, it's best (sorry to say) not to meditate in your comfortable reclining lounge chair.

Next, pick a regular time to meditate every day. Make it a top priority in your life. Commit yourself to meditating on a regular basis. You may want to think of your meditation session as a daily appointment with God and Jesus, as I do, and keep that appointment without fail. I devote the early morning before sunrise to meditation, as well as the early evening. This process of bookending my day with the disciplined practice helps me start and end the day on a peaceful, positive note. If you can, choose a quiet time of day for meditating. Earplugs or noise-reducing headphones are sometimes helpful.

If you aren't comfortable sitting on the floor, select a chair where you can sit with your spine straight—posture is important. It's mentioned earlier, but bears repeating: the chair seat should be flat and parallel to the ground. Sitting with your back and neck straight, not supported by the chair's back, will make the energy flow more easily through your spine. Find a position you can sit in fairly comfortably without slumping. Lying down is not recommended because it encourages falling asleep.

As in any physical activity, it is better to begin with brief sessions of meditating and develop a regular practice than it is to start by sitting for hours at a time and then give up in frustration. I recommend starting with 10 to 15 minutes once a day. In the beginning it is most important to establish a regular time for meditation and to stick with it. Later you may want to meditate more frequently or for greater lengths of time.

Regardless of the technique you use, you'll find that the mind wanders and the body experiences unusual sensations. Most traditions recommend that you not try to avoid thinking or being distracted. When you realize you are distracted, gently bring your mind back to its object of concentration. Each time the mind wanders and is brought back, your ability to concentrate has been strengthened. Your mind is being trained to respond to you, rather than being allowed to lead you according to its whims. Let's say you have chosen to focus on your breath as you slowly and deeply inhale and exhale. The minute you become aware that you're not focusing on your breath, gently but firmly refocus on it. Through this process of focusing and refocusing on one point, your internal "noise" eventually diminishes; your mind is quieter, and your energy level is higher.

Deeper levels of meditation begin after the initial noise and distracting thoughts have been cleared away. Usually, periods of quiet, when it's easy to focus, alternate with periods of unintentional random thinking. As you continue to meditate, the times of easier focus, greater clarity, and inner quiet lengthen. These periods of quiet joyfulness are the first goal of meditation. There is no limit to the depth, energy, and peacefulness that can be achieved in meditation.

Each session of meditation should be continued until a quiet mental state is reached. Don't stop in the middle of a lot of thoughts, when you're having difficulty concentrating. Wait until a time when you are quiet, then stop.

> There is no limit to the depth, energy, and peacefulness that can be achieved in meditation.

The periods of noise and quiet will alternate as your meditation breaks through layers of thoughts and tension. You will feel renewed if you can stop after reaching any still place; it isn't necessary to reach samadhi (bliss) to have a great meditation.

Even though the goal is absolute quiet, it's important to start your sessions with your energy as high as possible. It's nice to have showered first, or at least to feel awake. The more alert and energized you feel, the easier it will be to focus and meditate. It's also best to meditate on an empty stomach, and definitely not after eating a heavy meal.

Don't be too rigid in your practice. On occasion, find other special places to meditate. I often become immersed in meditation in the outdoors—at the beach, in the mountains, or in a nearby park. I welcome the sounds of nature when I meditate outdoors. Being out in nature encourages mindfulness, helping you to see and hear things more clearly and become one with your surroundings.

Nature Meditation

In Joseph Cornell's book *Listening to Nature*, I learned about a nature meditation he refers to as "stillness meditation." It combines concentrative and mindfulness elements. Here's the technique, which I sometimes practice while out in nature. It helps to quiet restless thoughts and sometimes brings wonderful calmness.

❖ First, relax the body: Do this by inhaling and tensing all over—feet, legs, back, arms, neck, face—as much as you possibly can. Then exhale and relax completely. Repeat this several times.

❖ To practice the technique itself: Observe the natural flow of your breath. Do not control the breath in any way! Simply follow it attentively. Each time you inhale, think "still." Each time you exhale, think "ness." Repeating "still . . . ness" with each complete breath helps focus your mind on the present moment and keeps your attention from wandering.

❖ During the pauses between inhalation and exhalation: Stay in the present moment, calmly observing whatever is in front of you. If thoughts of the past or future disturb your mind, just calmly and patiently bring your attention back to what is before you, and to repeating "still . . . ness" with your breathing.

Stillness meditation, explains Cornell, "will help you to become absorbed in natural settings for longer and longer periods. Use it when you want to feel this calmness, indoors or outdoors, with eyes open or closed."

White Light Meditation

The following kind of meditation, called White Light meditation, is one that can be done anywhere and is easy for beginners as well as advanced students of meditation.

1. Sit in a straight-backed chair with spine erect and feet flat on the floor. (You can also sit cross-legged on the floor if you wish.) Fold your hands together in your lap, or hold them in prayer position. Eyes may be open or closed.

2. Feel yourself relaxing as you take several long, slow, deep breaths.

3. Imagine a beautiful white light glowing from within and completely surrounding you. This is your protection as you open sensitive energy centers, and you can use this with any of your meditations.

4. For about 10 minutes, gently concentrate on a single idea, picture, or word. Select something that is meaningful, uplifting, and spiritual to you. (I choose to focus on Jesus.) You might even focus on some peaceful music.

5. If your mind wanders from your object of focus, gently bring it back to what you are concentrating on.

6. After 10 minutes, separate your hands and turn them palms up in your lap. If your eyes have been closed, open them.

7. Relax your focus on the object of concentration and shift your mind into neutral.

8. Remain passive, yet alert, for 10 more minutes. Gently observe any thoughts and images that may float by. Just be still and detached, and remain present with whatever you are experiencing.

This 20-minute meditation recharges your energy field and nourishes creativity and tranquility. At other times during the day, allow the same sensation of light to flow from within your being, and let it fill your entire body. It's very easy to do, and it puts you into a meditative state.

If you prefer guided relaxation meditations, I have recorded six different pieces as part of my audio program *Celebrate Life!*, which incorporates music and nature sounds. I also have another meditation in my audio program *Wired to Meditate*.

Susan's Favorite Christian Meditations

From the Bible, I have selected some of my favorite passages. For example, in **Psalm 46:10**, we read. "Be still and know that I am God." So, I have taken that passage and gently created the phrase of "Peace . . . Be Still." Many of my meditations use this phrase, and when I slowly and deeply inhale, I say silently to myself, "Peace." I'll hold my breath for 3 or more seconds, and then when I exhale, I say "be still." These three simple words bring me deep relaxation and calmness as I imagine Jesus is saying the words to me.

I also use the phrase "In Thee . . . I Trust" and I'll inhale to "In Thee" and exhale to the words "I Trust."

Similarly, I will take the words "I AM" and inhale to these two powerful words, and then add on an adjective for the exhalation phase that fits my personal goals or desires on that day. In other words, if I am feeling stressed out on a particular day, I might do a meditation with inhalation and exhalation and repeat slowing and gently, I AM (inhale) . . . calm (exhale) or I AM . . . serene, I AM . . . peace; or maybe even I AM . . . tranquil. The three dots indicate the slow, deep, and deliberate breaks between the inhalation and the exhalation.

If my self-esteem and confidence need to be bolstered, I would meditate on "I AM . . . valuable" or I AM . . . deserving," etc. Select any adjectives that support your goals in every area of your life. Here's are some adjectives from which to choose: I AM . . . healthy; I AM . . . confident; I AM . . . kind; I AM . . . creative; I AM . . . fit and strong; I AM . . . successful; I AM . . . prosperous; I AM . . . accepted; I AM . . . content; I AM . . . victorious; I AM . . . triumphant; I AM . . . forgiven; I AM . . . grateful; I AM . . . blessed; I AM . . . God-centered; I AM . . . God's child; I AM . . . divinely guided; and one of my favorite adjectives . . . I AM . . . wonderful. I also use often, I AM renewed and . . . restored in God.

Two of my favorite deep breathing, meditative, and prayerful affirmations are also "Be still and know" (inhale slowly and deeply to those four words) ". . . that I AM God" (exhale slowly to those four words) again from **Psalm 46:10**.

The other one is this: "I AM a child . . . of the . . . Most High God." On this one, I inhale to the words "I AM a child," and then I gently hold my breath for the words "of the," followed by exhaling to the words "Most High God." I will often do this slowly and resolutely for several minutes. What's more, this powerful, positive, and life-affirming phrase is often what I will repeat when waiting in line at the grocery store, post office, or other location, when I'm putting gas in my car, when hiking in the mountains or walking on the beach, and even as part of my grace before my meals. With gratitude to God and Jesus is always the intent in my heart when I repeat any of these affirmations. In fact, at the end of all of my meditations, I say silently or out loud, "In the name of Jesus, thank you, praise be to God. Amen."

There's no limit to how often you can repeat this **Psalm 46:10** daily and in any situation. The affirmative blessings that this meditative prayer will contribute to your life will amaze you, even if it's only a few minutes a day. As a result, you will experience an increase in your confidence, self-esteem, faith, hope, peace, prosperity, as well as appreciate more balance in your life. I often refer to this as my "Magnet for Blessings" meditative prayer because it results in triumph for everyone who recites it often.

Action Step

At least a few times daily, for one month, just 30 days, I encourage you to do this breathing affirmation and notice the rewarding changes in your life. You've got nothing to lose and everything to gain.

It was my grandmother who taught me about the power of the words I AM when I was a teenager and how to construct these positive affirmations. Then, in 2015, David Craddock gifted me with a copy of Joel Osteen's inspiring book entitled *The Power of I AM*. This book covers in detail how to use I AM to help you create your best life. In Chapter 1 of his book, Joel writes this:

> Rather than being down on ourselves and discrediting who we are and focusing on all of our flaws, I wonder what would happen if all through the day—not in front of other people, but in private— we were to be as bold as David [from the Bible] was and say, "I am amazing. I am wonderful. I am valuable." When you talk like that, amazing comes chasing you down. Awesome starts heading in your direction. You won't have that weak, defeated, "I'm just average" mentality. You'll carry yourself like a king, like a queen. Not in pride. Not being better than somebody, but with a quiet confidence, with the knowledge that you've been handpicked by the Creator of the universe.

I AM ... grateful—that you are reading this book and joining me in upgrading our lives. Together let's enjoy the blessings from doing these I AM affirmations daily.

Spiritual Blessings from Meditation

The longer any individual practices meditation, the greater the likelihood that his or her goals and efforts will shift toward personal and spiritual growth. As I travel around the country and world giving talks and meeting people, it delights me to learn how many people are taking responsibility for their health and lives and embracing a holistic program that includes meditation. It's not uncommon for me to hear: "I began meditating to decrease my stress and to feel a sense of control in my life. But as my practice deepens, not only do I feel more relaxed, I also am developing a more open heart—more sensitivity, greater compassion, less negative judgment toward others, and a deeper relationship with God and Jesus."

Many individuals who initially learn meditation for its self-regulatory aspects find that as their practice deepens they are drawn more and more into the realm of the spiritual. Meditation is all about breaking out of the everyday world of tensions and thoughts and finding the place of inner peace, calmness, insight, and enlightenment. It will change your life because it changes you. Find the method or methods that suit you best.

As a part of creating vibrant health, our goal must be to integrate spirituality into every area of our lives. The essence of who we are is pure Spirit; we bring it with us in everything we think, feel, say, and do. An 18-inch journey from your head to your heart keeps you open to Spirit's presence. In other words, jettison judgmental, critical, and the-world-centers-around-me type of thinking in favor of being more tenderhearted, as I wrote about in Chapter 2. This takes discipline, courage, and a warrior's strength. It's not for the faint of heart or the weak-minded. In his book, *A Path with Heart*, Jack Kornfield writes from a similar perspective:

We need energy, commitment, and courage not to run from our life nor to cover it over with any philosophy—material or spiritual. We need a warrior's heart that lets us face our lives directly, our pains and limitations, our joys and possibilities. This courage allows us to include every aspect of life in our spiritual practice: our bodies, our families, our society, politics, the Earth's ecology, art, education. Only then can spirituality be truly integrated into our lives.

In her work with many cancer and AIDS patients, Dr. Borysenko has observed that many people are interested in meditation as a way of becoming more attuned to the spiritual dimension of life. She reports that many patients die "healed," in a state of compassionate self-awareness and self-acceptance.

Quiet your mind in meditation to experience the perfect rhythm of the universe. When you go within, jettison negative and judgmental thoughts, and allow yourself the freedom to be at peace by simply meditating and experiencing the oneness of all life, you soon start to find that energy which is blissful and enlightening. If meditation is practiced enough, that quiet mind state will convince you of the oneness and perfection of everything.

Although we may look different on the outside, we are all one in spirit with God and with one another, and we share the same innate spirituality. It's hard to remember this truth in today's tumultuous world. When we watch the TV or go online to read magazines or newspapers, it's easy to forget that we're all made of the same stuff, so much more alike than different. By meditating and following God's Light and Love within us, we can naturally live together in peace and harmony. If we are faced with or witnessing intolerance from others, meditation can give us strength to bless the situation and acknowledge that there is a Divine Power in charge. Obstacles are what we see when we take our eyes off the vision and

> Quiet your mind in meditation to experience the perfect rhythm of the universe.

separate ourselves from one another. Although others may seem worlds apart from us, the acceptance we feel in meditation reminds us that we all look at the same sky, bask in the glow of the same sun, and are blessed by the same intelligence and omnipresence that guides the universe. Meditation helps keep our heart connected to God and our eyes focused on our vision.

The Divine Surrender

During my meditation period, I often incorporate visualization, affirmations, and prayer, and most often my prayer involves surrender to God. What is it that I surrender? Negative feelings, negative thoughts, fears, resentments, addictions, and resistance.

> *Resistance to change is nothing more*
> *than hardening of the attitudes.*

Through studying the Bible and the words of Jesus, I understand the power of surrender. I will often say this silently to myself or out loud: "Lord, I am your child; during good and difficult times. I love You. You are with me always guiding me in everything I think, feel, say, and do." In that prayer of perfect surrender, I feel my life to be in a Divine embrace, living from the Christ-Light within me and know that everything is unfolding perfectly in my life.

Surrender brings with it gratitude. Gratitude, an overflowing feeling of thanksgiving, is the instant response of the soul touched by awareness of the Divine, of God. With even a momentary awakening to God's Presence within, such joyous freedom bathes our consciousness and provides a blessed release from all the tensions and fears and anxieties that weigh us down in this world. In **1 Thessalonians 5:16-18** we read:

> *16 Rejoice always, 17 pray continually,*
> *18 give thanks in all circumstances;*
> *for this is God's will for you in Christ Jesus.*

Surrender means letting go, trusting in the forces and principles that are always at work in the universe, and living with spiritual elegance. With surrender comes an inner knowing and contentment. With surrender we can see the perfection of life and accept the paradox that all the suffering in the world is a part of that perfection, as is our own strong desire to help end it. One positive way to surrender is to make a personal commitment to forgive every single person with whom we have ever had any conflict, starting with ourselves. Brook no interference in this process of forgiveness, as it will transform and enrich your life in miraculous ways. Your resplendent inner Christ will shine through and serenity will become your joyful companion.

Choosing to forgive unlocks the gate to healing and health, prosperity and abundance, joy and happiness, and inner peace. Forgiveness is integral to the teachings of Jesus. Through the teachings of the Bible, He teaches us how forgiveness can heal our minds, dispel our pain, and ultimately awaken us from the confines of time and space. Jesus is pure Love and when we surrender to Him, love and forgiveness become the essence of our being, and forgiveness is the vehicle that helps us to release fear. Through forgiveness, miracles occur.

Medical researchers are also coming to the conclusion that an unforgiving nature may be one of the major culprits in human disease. One researcher calls arthritis "bottled hurt." If we condemn, criticize, or resent, or if we feel guilty, shameful, or angry toward another, we are only hurting ourselves. And until we practice forgiveness in our lives, the past will continue to repeat itself.

You become linked to another person when you don't offer forgiveness. You also give away your power and create a highly charged, emotionally active connection. But when you forgive, you take back your power and can no longer be controlled by the other person.

Some may say that forgiveness is a sign of weakness. I don't agree with that opinion. It takes strength and courage and a generous spirit to understand that people do not always hurt us because they choose to, but more likely because they couldn't help it or because we were in their way.

People do harm to others when they are in pain and are out of alignment with their Source, separated from God. If you give back to another person the same pain that person has given you, you are hurting yourself and making it impossible for a miracles to occur.

You can transform any negative emotion into love. While you can't control another person's feelings, you can choose what you want to experience and how you want to be. Let kindness and tenderheartedness be your goal. Jesus tells us to love our enemies. This is one of my favorite passages by Fred Rogers:

> *Imagine what our real neighborhoods would be like if each of us offered . . . just one kind word to another person.*
>
> ~FRED ROGERS

I understand how difficult this can be, especially when you believe someone has wronged you. Maybe you ask yourself, "How can I forgive what this person has done to me?" The secret is to get yourself out of the way and let Spirit forgive through you. When you choose to live your life more internally, allowing God to express His Light and Love through you, your heart softens and your life changes. Resentments, anger, guilt, and hurt are released. But you can't always release these negative emotions yourself. In my prayer time every day, I ask God to show me how to forgive the past, to forgive others, and to forgive myself.

Make meditation and prayer a top priority in your life. In time, and with disciplined practice, your life will become an expression of meditation and prayer, mindful and concentrated all the time. Meditation and prayer are the medium of miracles. When you meditate and pray daily, you can't not change. The joy you receive can be continuous.

Some of the prayers I say each day include:

 Lord, make me an instrument of peace and harmlessness.
I behold the Divine in everyone and everything.
I trust in Thee; show me the way.
God is in the driver's seat of my life.
Peace, be still, and know that I AM God.

The more you can love everything and everyone and feel gratitude for every moment, the healthier and more balanced your life will be.

The body benefits from movement, and the mind from stillness.
~SAKYONG MIPHAM

It is one of the most beautiful compensations of this life that no man can sincerely try to help another without helping himself. . . Serve and thou shall be served.
~RALPH WALDO EMERSON

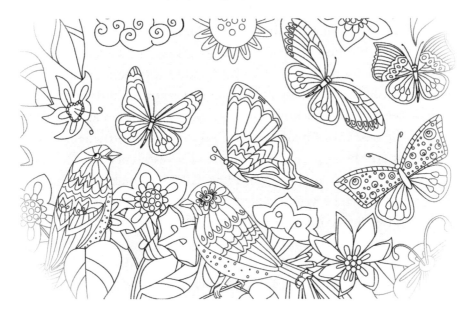

Chapter 9

Opening Up to Abundance & Blessings

It's God's will for you to live in prosperity instead of poverty.
It's God's will for you to pay your bills and not be in debt.

~JOEL OSTEEN

If the human race wishes to have a prolonged and indefinite
period of material prosperity, they have only got to behave
in a peaceful and helpful way toward one another.

~WINSTON CHURCHILL

One of the workshops and lectures I offer around the world is titled "Choose to Be Prosperous." In these presentations, I cover the topics of creating high-level wellness, attracting abundance and prosperity, and living with calm self-assurance, among many other subjects. On a number of occasions, I invited David Craddock to be a guest speaker at my workshops to talk about "Investment Matters" and cover topics such as saving money, clearing up debt, teaching children about money, finding the best investment manager, preparing for retirement or college, what are the best and worst kinds of investments, how to invest wisely, and much more. David also knows how to make financial and investment principles very practical so that the workshop participants can use this valuable information in their lives immediately, and create more abundant and prosperous lifestyles beginning that same day.

So in this chapter, I will briefly cover some of the practical tips I offer in my prosperity workshops on how to thrive and get more into the vibration of wealth and vitality rather than lowering yourself to the vibration of "brokenness" and dis-ease.

The Vibration of Wealth & Life

First, let's clarify what I mean when I say the word *vibration*. This is not a New Age term; rather it has to do with physics. While I am not an expert in physics, over the last 20 years, I have read my fair share of physics books and am fascinated by the topic. Put simply, physics is the scientific study of matter and energy and how they interact with each other. This energy can take the form of motion, lights, electricity, radiation, gravity, and vibration—just about anything. Physics deals with matter on scales ranging from subatomic particles (i.e., the particles that make up the atom and the particles that make up *those* particles) to stars and even entire galaxies.

Every living thing is acting in a way that is fundamentally driven by the particles of which it is composed. You've probably heard the term *quantum physics*. In physics, quantum has to do with the quantity of energy proportional in magnitude to the frequency of the radiation it represents. (That's a mouthful and an interesting sentence to bring up at the next boring party you attend!) Quantum physics is the physics that governs the domain of the very, very small. Our brains have evolved to understand objects (from the size of ants to marine mammals as big as whales) going at medium speeds. When things go very fast or are very small, our minds don't comprehend this very well.

Science uses models to describe reality. One model of light is that it is a wave, sort of like a water wave. Another model is that it is a particle. Wave particle duality doesn't just exist for light. It's also true of atoms, electrons, and other particles. What I like to say in my workshops to make it all more understandable is that everything, down to the simplest level of existence, is light and movement and actually not solid. The chair you sit on, the bed you sleep on, and even your entire body, down to the simplest level is not really solid at all; it's a wave of energy and vibration, oscillations.

Take food, for example. Foods have different levels of vibration. Organic fruits and vegetables (sun foods) have a higher level of vibration than animal products like beef and chicken. When you take the colorful produce into your body, it actually increases the vibrational rate of the electrons and atoms in your body. That's a good thing! You always want to increase the vibrational rate of your body. Positive thinking increases the vibrational rate; so does meditation, beautiful music, and spending time outdoors in nature. Being grateful increases the overall vibrational rate in your body.

All of your thoughts either increase or decrease the vibrational rate of your body. When you think high vibrational thoughts such as focusing on those things for which you are grateful and looking for things to appreciate, you add to the positive overall vibration of your body. On the flipside, however, when your thoughts are continually negative, or you focus on how you don't have the money to pay your bills, or you don't like how you look and more, all of this lowers the overall vibrational rate of your body and often leads to depression.

Since your time may be limited, let me get to the point of vibration and abundance. If you want to create a prosperous life, you must get into the vibration of wealth and synchronize all of your thoughts, words, and actions in support of your goal—creating a life filled with vitality, prosperity, and equanimity. In other words, be aware of your thoughts, the words you speak, and the actions you take and make sure they all support your goal of a spectacular life.

I've discussed these 12 tips with David on numerous occasions and he agrees with them all. We are both advocates of positive thinking and only putting out into the world, in thoughts, words, and actions, what we want to create in our lives. *This adds to the positive vibration.* Focusing on negativity—or what you don't want in your life—brings more of the same back into your life. In other words, what we think about, we bring about. We always attract to ourselves the equivalency of what we think, say, and do. And as my Danish grandmother, Fritzie, always used to say to me, *"Your attitude is your mind's paintbrush; it can color anything."* It starts in your mind with what you think moment to moment. Think thoughts of abundance, prosperity, and wealth, and only how you want your life to be—not the opposite.

12 Tips to Vibrate at a Higher Level
So Wealth Flows to You and Not Away from You

As you'll undoubtedly agree, it's necessary these days to have money so that your basic needs can be covered—freeing you to work on more important things, such as your health and essential spiritual matters. To help you thrive with success, here are some suggestions to get into the money vibration that I cover in my workshops, during radio interviews worldwide, and in more detail in my book *Choose to Thrive*. These 12 tips will neutralize the vibration of lack and introduce the vibration of wealth into your being and life.

1 SHARE WHAT YOU HAVE. To get into the wealth vibration, start sharing with people what you already have, even if you have very little at the moment. This sharing action will affirm to your mind that you have so much wealth that you can even share it.

One powerful way to increase your abundance is through tithing. Tithing traditionally means to give a tenth of your income to your church, but tithing doesn't necessarily have to go to a church—and it doesn't have to be 10 percent. Tithe gifts can be in monetary form or a giving of yourself in time and/or deposits of love. I tithe money to my church and to those who feed my soul and nourish me spirituality and who are making a positive difference on this planet, whether they are individuals or organizations. I also give money and time to people less fortunate than I. Remember, though, it's futile to say, "Yes, when such-and-such money comes in, I will give a tenth of it as a tithe." You have to start helping those in need before that, acting in the spirit of "give that you may receive."

One day, after writing my prosperity affirmations and goals on cards, I went to the grocery store. While waiting in the checkout line, I suddenly called out to the harried mother with two crying babies in front of me who didn't have enough to cover all of her groceries, "I'll pay for those." Needless to say, she was astonished! Quite honestly, so was I; the words seemed to have just popped out of my mouth. After some hesitancy on her part and some impressive cajolery on mine, she let me pay her bill. The pleasure I received made me feel rich inside. Later that same day, I ran into a person whom I had counseled several months before. At that time she had been unable to pay, and I had written the sessions off as a good learning experience. This day, seemingly out of the blue, she wrote me a check for twice the amount she owed me, saying that my guidance had a profound, positive effect on her life. So find ways today and every day to share what you have with others and notice how good it makes you feel.

2 FREE YOURSELF FROM DEBT. You must get out of debt, even if you need to sell some of your personal belongings for it, and never get back into debt. Debt enslaves you to the person or institution you owe and locks you into the vibration of lack and helplessness. And, of course, you must never live beyond your means. Have a monthly budget and stick to it.

3 BE AWARE OF WHAT YOU SAY–THE WORDS YOU SPEAK. Stop talking negatively about your financial situation. Complaining about it again locks you into this negative vibration. Only talk about your finances if you have something positive to say about it, for example, if your money situation is improving. Repeat daily over and over these two powerful prosperity affirmations—both out loud and also silently to yourself:

"I am connected to an unlimited source of abundance."

"I bless and prosper everyone in my life and everyone in my life blesses and prospers me."

And then live as though these affirmations are both true in your life—because they are! For more information on the healing power of affirmations, your words and thoughts and how to create your highest vision, please refer to my books *Choose to Thrive* and *Affirming God's Love*.

4 LET GO OF WORRY. This may be much easier said than done, but I know you can do it. Stop worrying about money, comfort, security, and other material things. How do you do this? If you stop worrying about such matters by increasing your faith in God, you will find that you become a magnet for prosperity. As I mentioned earlier in the book, one of my favorite quotes on faith is by Ralph Waldo Trine who wrote, *"Faith is an invisible and invincible magnet, and attracts to itself whatever it fervently desires and persistently expects."*

5 HEALTH BEFORE WEALTH. It was Ralph Waldo Emerson who once wrote this: *"Health is our greatest wealth."* I have certainly found this to be true in my life. You must grow in vibrant health before you can attract and hold on to your wealth. The healthier you are, the more confident and empowered you become, and this attracts wealth to you. In other words, without your health, it's very difficult to grow wealthy. If you have a hard time getting out of bed in the morning because you are exhausted; if you have ailments and health issues dragging you down; if you look and feel years older than your age; if you are sick and tired of being sick and tired; then take care of this immediately. Do what needs to be done to get healthy, fit, and vibrant. If you need help, please refer some of my other books mentioned at the beginning of this book.

6 PAY ATTENTION AND BE MINDFUL. Observe nature to learn the lessons it has about abundance. Everything in nature happens effortlessly and the manifestations of abundance are everywhere. Look at the sky and see a group of birds flying; look at the ground and see countless ants working; look at the trees to observe an abundance of lush leaves moving with the breeze. Train your eye this way to focus on abundance everywhere, rather than lack, and this way your mind will manifest abundance in your life, too. If all you did was just look for things to appreciate, your level of abundance would skyrocket and you would live a joyous, wonderful life.

EXPAND YOUR CONSCIOUSNESS
TO ATTRACT EVEN MORE

For more in-depth, life-enriching information that can help you live a fuller life, consider my special audio package entitled *Calm, Cool & Collected*, which is available on my website. In addition to becoming upwardly mobile, you will experience a fuller, happier, and more balanced life as you put the principles provided into practice.

7 GUARD YOUR THOUGHTS. Don't accept lack statements from the people you know. Especially if you live with people who have a vibration of lack, learn to guard your mind against their harmful statements. For example, if someone says to you, *"You will never be able to buy a car or the home of your dreams,"* reject their words immediately. When someone says something like that, don't accept those words as seeds in the soil of your mind, and instead affirm something positive, in the present tense and as though it's already your reality like this: *I am living in my beautiful home, paid in full, and driving my new car. I always have an abundance of money to create a wonderful life and to share with others."* This will make your mind strong, and it will be able to resist being dragged down into the lower vibrations.

8 MEDITATE ON FLOWING WATER. Meditate on the sounds of flowing water, such as a river or a babbling brook: The flow of water is the representation of the flow of money. Keep this observation in mind, only this one thought, when observing the flowing water. In my office and home, I have a small audio device that plays different sounds of nature. One of them is the sound of a mellifluous babbling brook, and I often turn this on to relax me and to hear the sound of flowing water. Even on my website, I have a variety of calming sounds of nature you can listen to. During my meditation sessions, I will sometimes turn on these nature sounds and find it very soothing and peaceful. You can also bring a small water fountain into your home so you are always surrounded by nature sounds and the flow of water.

9 **SPEND YOUR MONEY WISELY.** Spend money to make money. Even though you may have very little money currently, learn to spend it wisely. At this stage of lack, it's vitally important for you to put the roots of money multiplication into your being. You can do that by investing your money to make more money. Maybe you invest it to monetize an idea or business concept, keep money in a bank account with a good interest rate, or buy something like a washing machine or a lawnmower for other people to rent. This will not only multiply your money, but will also teach a valuable lesson of passive income.

10 **RESPECT YOUR MONEY–PAPER, COINS, AND CREDIT CARDS.** Don't simply throw your money into your wallet, purse, or other receptacle. Money needs to be respected. Always keep it aligned without creased corners, wadded up, or messy. I even take this a step further. In my wallet, my paper bills are all lined up and put in descending order and all facing the same direction. For example, my wallet might have one 100-dollar bill, two 50-dollar bills, followed by three 20-dollar bills, followed by two 10-dollar bills, followed by three 5-dollar bills, and, lastly, three 1-dollar bills. Keep your credit cards in alignment, too, and have as your goal to pay them off *in full* monthly, or at least every 90 days. If my money gets too old, I make a visit to the bank to trade it in for new money. If you respect your money in this simple, yet practicable way, it will return the favor by multiplying and growing for you.

Here's a quick example of how this played out for one of my friends. Sarah called me up and asked if she could take me to lunch in Brentwood (Los Angeles) near where I live because she needed some of my prosperity guidance. A year earlier, she had taken my workshop "Choose to Thrive: Steps to Creating a More Balanced Lifestyle." I hadn't seen her in about five months. Over lunch, she told me that a month prior, they phased out her job at her company so she was out of work. And after sending out multiple résumés to different companies, she hadn't gotten so much as a nibble of interest from anyone. She was at a loss for what to do next. When our lunch bill arrived, she took out her wallet, opened it up, and wrinkled paper money was falling out all over the table. The bills were creased, ripped, folded, and a total mess. I reminded Sarah that in my workshop a year prior, I taught everyone the importance of treating our money with respect and then it would grow for us, and even showed them my tips on organizing one's wallet. She admitted that this key point was the one thing she hadn't done yet. So I said that there's no better time than the present, and together we organized all the money in her tattered wallet.

Next, I excused myself, saying I was going to use the restroom and, instead, went next door to a lovely gift shop and purchased a beautiful new wallet for Sarah to hold all of her unwrinkled and organized money. Before I gave it to her, I reached into my wallet and pulled out a new $50 bill and slipped it into her wallet. When I gave her the present, she was overjoyed and so grateful. She loved the wallet in her favorite teal color (and even said she admired it before I arrived for lunch in the gift shop window and wished she could buy it) and even told me that this gift shop was her favorite store in Brentwood. In fact, three years earlier, I learned that she had applied for a job to be manager at the store but someone else got the position. We talked for about two more hours while sipping tea and I shared with her again some of the prosperity and health suggestions I've included in this chapter and in my books *Be the Change, Affirming God's Love*, and *Choose to Thrive*.

Well, that's not the end of the story. After I treated Sarah to lunch, we went together to the gift shop and looked around. While she was trying on scarves, I was near the front counter and overheard the store's manager on the telephone telling someone that she needed to find a replacement for her position because her husband just got a promotion and new job in another state and they needed to move quickly. I rushed over to Sarah to share with her what I heard and she was gobsmacked and a little nervous at the idea of talking to this manager about the position. We walked over together and I told the manager that I couldn't help overhearing her news about moving, and Sarah told her she would like to apply for this position again. This store manager was now also astonished at how quickly everything was happening. It turns out that Sarah got the job that same day, the manager was able to move quickly without worrying about how to find a replacement, and I was delighted that everyone was so happy.

Okay, I know what you are thinking. Did simply organizing the unwrinkled bills (showing great respect to the money) in the new wallet get Sarah the new job? We won't really ever know for sure, but I've seen things like this happen too many times to refute it as just a coincidence. You must always respect your money and how you carry it in your wallet, and it will respect you by growing and multiplying.

It's also a great lesson to learn about timing and how we are always at the right place at the right time. If we arrived only a couple minutes later at the gift shop, I would not have heard the manager on the telephone talking about needing to find someone to replace her quickly. Trust more and live with faith. As I mentioned earlier, have faith that everything is working for your highest good. Trust that all the unexpected changes in your daily and weekly schedule are a result of God making the necessary adjustments to help your days and life unfold in Divine Order.

And, yes, I now get to visit Sarah more often during her breaks from the gift shop at our favorite restaurant in Brentwood. She never lets me pay for lunch anymore when we meet at the restaurant next to the gift shop, which, by the way, is now doing better than ever before since Sarah is at the helm.

11 BALANCE YOUR MIND WITH DEEP BREATHING AND QUIET YOUR THOUGHTS. This might sound strange to you, but I've seen this one special tip work miracles in people lives. Balance your body and mind with deep breathing so that you will feel stable, self-assured, and attuned to the material money vibration inside you, if having more money is your goal. I also focus on the many quotes in the Bible about prosperity, such as **Deuteronomy 1:11, Deuteronomy 8:18, Deuteronomy 28:11, Deuteronomy 29:9, Deuteronomy 30:9, Philippians 4:19,** and **2 Chronicles 31:21.** By not providing the passages for you here, I have encouraged you to check these out yourself.

I might also focus on the many quotes from the masters of the past that I have collected over the years on prosperity, success, life, happiness, and balanced living such as these 10 favorites of mine by Ralph Waldo Emerson: *1) Do not go where the path may lead, go instead where there is no path and leave a trail; 2) Write it on your heart that every day is the best day of the year; 3) What lies behind you and what lies in front of you pales in comparison to what lies inside of you; 4) Nature always wears the colors of the spirit; 5) To be yourself in a world that is constantly trying to make you something else is the greatest accomplishment; 6) Never lose an opportunity of seeing anything beautiful, for beauty is God's handwriting; 7) Adopt the pace of nature: her secret is patience; 8) Once you make a decision, the universe conspires to make it happen; 9) Nothing great was ever achieved without enthusiasm; 10) The age of a woman doesn't mean a thing. The best tunes are played on the oldest fiddles.* Who doesn't love the sagacity and perspicacity of the one and only Ralph Waldo Emerson? And, yes, ladies, we are all magnificent fiddles!

You can learn more about deep breathing and meditation and how to do this, as well as holistic health in general, in my audio programs *Choose to Live Peacefully* and *Wired to Meditate*.

12 BE AFFLUENT AND PROSPEROUS IN ALL WAYS. Replace cheap stuff with wealth-affirming items in your home. It's better, for example, to have fewer good-quality clothes than many cheap things to wear. Everything in your surroundings affirms whether you are wealthy or poor, so make sure that, at least, your home is the symbol of abundance rather than lack. Make a commitment to excellence in your life and this includes what you wear, how you live, and what your home looks like.

And speaking of your home, here's my final tip. Make sure your home is an enjoyable place to be and live. We all need a sanctuary in life, a place of refuge and protection, a place filled with love and peace where we can recharge our batteries, replenish our souls, and then go out into the world and create great things. For most of us, this place is our home.

What can you do today to honor some or all of these suggestions? Here are prosperity affirmations to memorize and repeat often:

- *God's wealth and abundance are circulating in my life.*

- *I am connected to an unlimited source of abundance.*

- *In everything I do, I prosper.*

For countless more suggestions on using affirmations to create your best life, please refer to my book *Affirming God's Love*.

Never forget that you are the president and CEO of your body and life. You can create your best life and live with an abundance of joy, vibrant health, and happiness. If you would like any extra help with motivation to keep you on track, please refer to my books. All these tips will help you to raise your vibration to that of success, and open you up to a life filled and running over with vitality, prosperity, and success.

To me, prosperity is having health, having great children, having peace, good relationships. It's not about the money.

~JOEL OSTEEN

A man is not rightly conditioned until he is a happy, healthy, and prosperous being; and happiness, health, and prosperity are the result of a harmonious adjustment of the inner with the outer of the man with his surroundings.

~JAMES ALLEN

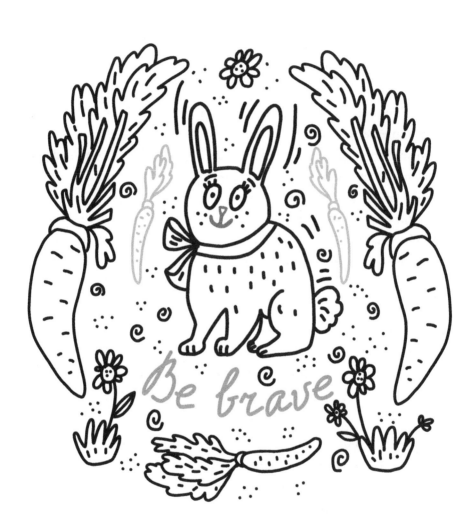

Be brave

Part 4

Profound Ways to Foster a Halcyon Life

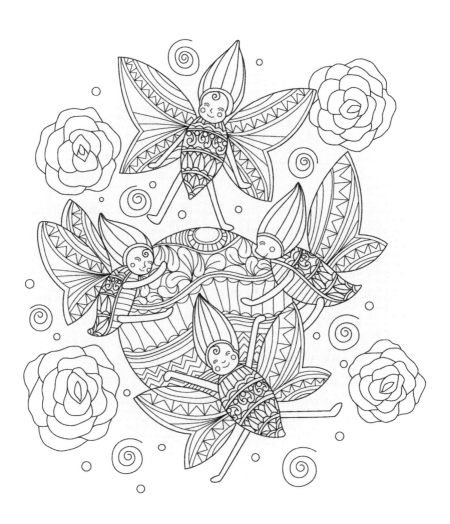

Chapter 10

Inviting Your
Inner Child to Play &
Help Orchestrate Your Day

*Cannot we let people be themselves,
and enjoy life in their own way?*

~Ralph Waldo Emerson

*The most wasted day of all is that
on which we have not laughed.*

~Sébastien Nicolas de Chamfort

When we are anchored in God, no matter what comes our way, we can remain positive and look for the good in everything. Easier said than done, right? Attitude makes all the difference. A positive attitude doesn't just happen by itself; we must cultivate it. William James, the noted philosopher, put it beautifully when he said that the greatest discovery of our generation is that a human being can alter his life by altering his attitude.

Indeed, situations will arise in our lives that may seem unpleasant or difficult, but a positive attitude sees problems as opportunities for growth. I believe that nothing happens in life that does not afford us the opportunity to deepen our understanding of and appreciation for life.

With your new positive attitude, you will come to understand that it is not the times, complications of society, or other people that cause problems. It is only your inability to cope. Whatever is going on with you at the moment, choose to make it okay. Give up the fear of making mistakes and the need for approval from others. Be yourself. I see so many people living according to how others expect them to be. This just leads to unhappiness. Live more from inner guidance, from God's whispering inside you. Understand that there is no absolute way to happiness. Rather, happiness is the way.

A negative attitude acts like an insulator that inhibits the flow of creative energy. Criticism, gossip, anger, fear, envy, suspicion, jealousy, worry, hate, doubt, laziness, anxiety, guilt, and shame are all forms of negative thinking. Watch your thoughts. Make them obey you. Train your mind to think constructively and positively at all times. A joyful, thankful attitude will carry you a long way toward the goal of bringing into your life the health, happiness, and peace that you desire and deserve.

It's been my experience that if you laugh and smile more, your attitude will tilt toward the positive. And if, by chance, you feel you don't have any reason to smile, let me give you four: It firms your facial muscles; it makes you feel better; it makes people wonder what you've been up to; and it is the shortest distance between two people.

And here's a fifth reason from Mother Teresa: "A smile is the beginning of peace."

Young children are my greatest teachers on how we can all enjoy and celebrate life. They laugh, tell jokes, play, sing, dance, move, and live in their own magical world.

Humor and laughter have both been found to be important components of healing and being radiantly healthy. William Fry of Stanford University has reported that laughter aids digestion, stimulates the heart, strengthens muscles, activates the brain's creative function, and keeps you alert. So make up your mind to laugh and be happy. As Abraham Lincoln said, "Most folks are about as happy as they make up their minds to be."

Laughter also helps you to keep your life in better perspective. When you laugh at yourself, you learn to take yourself far less seriously. "Angels fly because they take themselves lightly," says an old Scottish proverb, which I mentioned in the previous *Intermission*. This is a lovely thought.

So with the right attitude, with joy in your heart, with a smile on your face, and a guard at the door of your mind, you can experience life as a great adventure, a celebration of the Holy Spirit manifested everywhere and in everyone. You'll come to realize that life is meant to live one day at a time with a childlike sense of wonder and expectancy. It's not too late to experience life fully. As long as you're breathing, it's never too late.

Being Childlike

So many of us are searching for the "fountain of youth," the secret that will enable us to live long and healthy lives. We have looked to special diets, supplements, and exercise. Yet the secret to living a quality life, full of aliveness and celebration, comes from within—from our attitudes, our expressions, our thoughts, and how we view ourselves and the world around us. Young children can often provide the keys to celebrating life. They are some of my greatest teachers. They express pure joy.

I marvel at the way young children can be real, sensitive, and open with each other. Living heart-to-heart seems to be so natural for them. There are no masks when they relate to each other. When children meet for the first time, they will often relate as if they were lifetime buddies.

Compare this to your response when meeting someone new. Are you trusting, comfortable, and enthusiastic? Or perhaps suspicious, reserved, and unwilling to be vulnerable? We reflect our individual attitudes and feelings about ourselves. Every day we have an opportunity to spread some joy in this world by how we relate to other people. It could be something as simple as being a good listener or offering a warm hug. The other person receives your joy and will naturally pass it along to others. It's so simple and yet so profound. What you give comes back multiplied.

To be childlike is to be innocent of all the strange, authoritarian ideas of what adulthood ought to be; to be trusting and straightforward;

to be honest and natural, free from the need to impress others. Being childlike means being more concerned with your experience of life than how you look to others. You do not have to give up being an adult in order to become more childlike. You do not have to become infantile or in the least bit irresponsible or unaccountable. The fully integrated person is capable of the harmonious blending of the adult and the child.

Think about the adults you most like to be with. I'll bet they are genuinely happy, joyful people. From joyfulness flows laughter, a sense of humanness, and silliness. Too many adults take themselves so seriously that they've forgotten how to look at the bright side of things. You don't always have to be orderly, rigid, serious, and adult-like. Learn to laugh, especially at yourself. Learn to have fun and be a little silly and crazy. In other words, lighten up. When you do this, the whole world will seem brighter and more beautiful.

Within each of us is a child waiting to come forth and express himself or herself more fully. What usually keeps us from getting in touch with the child within is our unwillingness to recognize and accept this child. It seems we often feel that since we're grownups, we have to act our age.

There is a lovely passage in the Bible (**Matthew 19:14**): "Let the children come to me, and do not hinder them; for to such belongs the kingdom of heaven." Young children live in their own heaven, no matter what their background, the language they speak, or where they live. Children's celebrations of life, passion, and joy are universal.

Once, while I was jogging in a park in Switzerland, I noticed several children playing a game that was new to me. Their parents and nannies were sitting quietly and mostly focusing on their cell phones or tablets, not talking or paying much attention to the children. The kids were having a fantastic time laughing, running, touching, being silly, and enjoying one another's company. It looked like so much fun. After watching for a few minutes, I felt compelled to join them. Through hand signals I asked if I could play, and an hour later I was exhausted. Although I couldn't speak their language, we laughed a whole lot. There was a special bonding and love, a respect and sharing that transcended the need for words. Laughter can be so freeing and so uniting at the same time.

The very next day, toward the end of my walk, I saw a boy and girl down on all fours, looking keenly at the ground next to a beautiful flowering tree. I stopped to see what was so captivating. In intermittent English, their mother told me that for nearly 30 minutes the two children had been engrossed in watching some ants as they made their journey from the tree to a scattering of breadcrumbs a few feet away. Then and there I got down on my hands and knees, too, and for several precious minutes I joined the children in their adventure, becoming totally involved with them and the ants. It was delightful.

Reflect a moment on your own experiences being around children. What are children like? How do you feel when you are with them? What qualities do they express to you? Before you read on, write down some words that would describe your favorite children. As you read over the list, ask yourself how many of these qualities are part of your personality. Which ones would you like to develop or reawaken?

When I wrote my list, here are some words that came to my mind. Children are:

* sanguine
* alert

* eager
* trusting

* persevering
* open

They are also:

* energetic
* cheerful
* caring

* playful
* sensitive
* friendly

* inquisitive
* vivacious

They are enthusiastic, playful, expressive, spontaneous, and natural. They laugh a lot and love to act silly and crazy. They are innocently loving and incredibly lovable.

Your list may contain other adjectives, but from my perspective, these positive childlike qualities are the guaranteed recipe for living fully.

My mom, June, used to always remind me of this: *The more you love, the more you're loved, and the lovelier you are.* How true that is! And it begins with you and your relationship with God. Commit to strengthening your connection with God and living a God-centered life, and through this loving relationship, you can shine more brightly and share your loving God-powered presence with others in your life and beyond.

As children grow older, they are strongly influenced by the behavior of their role models and the mores of their society. This influence provides all the more reason for us to model for children a playful, childlike way to be a responsible adult.

Learning to laugh with children is one way to recover the aliveness and spontaneity that are missing in our lives. Other ways of getting to our inner fountains of joy are simplifying our lives, slowing down, taking time to smell the flowers, talking to the animals, watching the clouds, and being with family and friends.

In my life, I have noticed that when my judgmental self rears its ugly head, I tend to be more controlling of people and situations instead of letting go and flowing with life. When I choose to release my desire to be in control and to live more from inner guidance, I notice that struggle dissipates and I feel more joyful and peaceful about myself and my life.

The more I pay attention to how children experience and embrace life, and the more I release my fears about being rejected and feeling uncertain, the better life becomes for me and for those people around me, because the gentle, tenderhearted me comes forth. As that happens, the dichotomies of my life soften. My work becomes play; my challenges become wonderful opportunities to learn and grow. My life takes on clarity and purpose as I move closer to becoming a master of the art of living.

According to the late American writer James Michener:

> The master of the art of living draws no distinction between his work and his play, his labor and his leisure, his mind and his body, his education and his recreation, his love and his religion.

He hardly knows which is which. He simply pursues his vision of excellence through whatever he is doing and leaves it to others to decide whether he is working or playing. To himself, he is always going both.

Make a point of doing something out of the ordinary each day that brings joy to others and to yourself. The results may surprise you. I love teddy bears. Often when I take long trips in my car, my bears accompany me. I also take one when I fly out of town. My bears help keep my inner child alive and happy. As well, I have a stuffed animal of a horse (being a lover of horses) that is always present in my car to accompany me when driving.

Children accept you totally for your good points and your not-so-good points, too. They don't care about differences in people, about different races, religions, or backgrounds. I feel that in a world in which so much conflict exists between people of different religions, races, and backgrounds, the best bridge to understanding, peace, and joy is built of love and forgiveness. When we reach out to another and offer unconditional love and forgiveness, as children do, joy and peace are the result.

Living well means putting a big emphasis on having some fun.
~Alexandra Stoddard

Bless the good-natured, for they bless everybody else.
~Thomas Carlyle

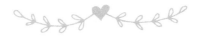

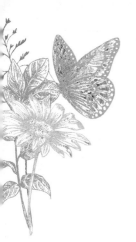

Chapter 11

Cultivating Courage
in Everything

Life is either a daring adventure—or nothing.

~Helen Keller

Live your life while you have it. Life is a splendid gift.

~Florence Nightingale

*I*t takes daring just to live, but it takes courage to live your vision. Is it possible to be in touch with your true courageousness without being in touch with your Divinity? I don't think so. We can soar to the top of the mountain and beyond when we know that the courage we want is part of us; it's our trust in Love, our trust in God. Trust in the Divine Loving Presence will destroy the fear that stifles our efforts.

Fear is our misperception of the situation. It's looking through our human eyes and mind rather than the eyes of the heart of God. When we face our fears, acting from the awareness that we are one with Spirit, we learn and nurture courage. Goethe said, "Whatever you can do, or dream you can, begin it. Boldness has genius, power, and magic in it." When we face our fears head-on, they begin to evaporate. When we embrace what scares us, we find that we are endowed with a level of courage that we never knew existed. Every day we have so many opportunities to act courageously. Committing to a new, upgraded healthy living program takes courage. Putting forth new and fresh ideas on paper each day takes courage. Getting up each morning to face the day as a willing and enthusiastic participant takes courage. Become enthusiastic about your life. Muster up the courage to live your life with gusto. It was Thomas Edison who said, "When a man dies, if he can pass enthusiasm along to his children, he has left them an estate of incalculable value."

Let courage be the shield that protects you. Let courage direct your spirit's light to shine on your path and give you strength to live your vision, to dare to risk, and go after your dreams. In the end, most people don't regret the things they do. They regret what they failed to do.

With so much negativity in the media and around the world these days, it takes courage to see the good and the positive. As you've probably read earlier in the book, I acquired the nickname "Sunny" because I always had a sunny disposition and, like Pollyanna, chose to look naïve, but I knew better. I saw the negative but chose to look beyond it, with the eyes of my heart.

Why do you defend your limitations? Why do you let fear paralyze you? You can choose differently. Instead, let God-Spirit (Light and Love) be your guide, with courage at the reins. Courage is going after the things you believe in even though they seem impossible.

Writer Louisa May Alcott, in her brilliant book *Little Women* (and the superb movie adaptation of the same name I saw in 2020), writes about how Jo March and her three sisters are determined to live life on their own terms during a time in our history when girls and women were not afforded the same opportunities as men and were encouraged to stay in the background of life and let men take the reins. I encourage you to read this book or enjoy the movie, especially if you are female. It's an inspiring story of living with courage and mettle.

My mom taught me to be courageous by being a shining example to me. She gave me the courage to believe I could do things I only dreamed of. She would never allow me to defend my limitations.

What is courage to you? To me, courage is moving through uncertainty. Courage is changing when that's the hardest thing in the world to do. Courage is being responsible for what you've created in your life and relinquishing blame. It's trusting in God when you want to be in charge. It's making difficult choices when, in this fast-paced, overstimulated world, we're overwhelmed with information. Courage is choosing to live peacefully and simply when everything in life seems to teach the opposite. Some people think that if you have courage, you don't have fear. Not at all! Courage is being fearful but doing it anyway, and courage is admitting you don't know.

Knowing that I would write the chapter on courage today, during my early morning hike, I thought more about this topic, and here are some other ideas that came to me. Courage is trusting again in a relationship, even when you've been hurt or disappointed. Courage is living up to the promises we've made to ourselves and to others. Courage is when we don't complain and we do what we have to do even though we might not want to. With courage, we move beyond ourselves.

I have had the pleasure of working with a variety of celebrities, CEOs, and world-class athletes through the decades and have talked with them on how they overcame their personal fears and, with courage, achieved their goals. What I learned from all of these encounters is that with courage, inner strength, belief, and faith, you can overcome any obstacle and make a difference in this world.

True courage enables us to live in the present moment and make choices rather than being a victim and settling for what life gives us. Sometimes we just need to make the choice to move in the direction of our dreams. Movement is powerful. Martha Graham, an American dancer and choreographer, a premier figure in modern dance who lived ninety-seven years, always advocated movement: "There is a vitality, a life force, an energy, a quickening that is translated through you into action, and because there is only one of you in all time, this expression is unique. And if you block it, it will never exist through any other medium and will be lost." I love that thought.

As I wrote about in the previous chapter on becoming more child-like, sometimes we overthink everything instead of living from trusting and simply being in the moment. Too much analyzing and rationalizing often leads to lack of courage. Let your inner child spark your motivation to take some action. I used to hear my friend Buckminster Fuller (Bucky, as I referred to him) say in his talks, "Dare to be naïve." Isn't that fantastic? You get an idea, it excites you, it makes you feel wonderful, it benefits you and others, it causes no harm to anyone, and it would be a joy to create in your life. Go for it. Do what it takes. Believe that you've been given this wish to fulfill and let no one and nothing cause you to doubt your power and ability to make this wish come true. Be just naïve enough to believe that this wish is yours to bring to fruition. Trust in the wish, take the steps necessary to bring it to fruition, and know that you deserve to create your best life. But it starts right here in the present moment.

Several years ago, I went to the Sierra Nevada Mountains alone for a few days of quiet, meditation, prayer, deep communion with God, and just being out in nature. On this particular summer trip, I had a cabin next to a placid, beautiful lake. The day before I came home, I decided to take an all-day hike in the mountains. I left at around dawn and hiked uphill for most of the morning. Around two in the afternoon, I decided to sit down, relax, and meditate by a tree. It was unusually quiet that day; I passed only five people on the trails. Sitting cross-legged, with my eyes still open, I could see paradise—several lakes and most of the Sierras. With each breath, I felt more peaceful, relaxed, and connected with God's healing light and love. I closed my eyes and began to concentrate on my breath, slowly inhaling and slowly exhaling. It felt wonderful. In a few more moments, I was totally absorbed in my inner world, not at all distracted by my surroundings, except for one minor thing. I thought I could hear some leaves moving. Often, when I'm meditating outdoors, I'm extra sensitive to nature's sounds. I figured I was in tune with the leaves and their musical dance. After a few more minutes, however, the sound of the leaves moving got louder. Slightly curious, I opened one eye. What I saw made my heart jump so that I thought it was on the outside of my body. No more than about 20 feet in front of me was a bear.

My first reaction was unbridled fear. The bear just stood there and stared at me. My second reaction was to ask God what to do. The answer was instant and, as I look back on the situation, somewhat off the wall. Or should I say off the tree? I was told to breathe slowly and deeply—as best I could, and stand up to make myself tall and scary to the bear. I was also told to smile at the bear and say some kind words from my heart. I gave it my best shot. I told the bear, in three octaves higher than I'm used to speaking, that he was beautiful, his fur was shiny, and that I didn't intend on being his lunch. By talking to him, I actually began to feel relaxed. As I acted with courage, the fear slowly began to disappear. For about five minutes, I spoke to the bear. Then something really amazing occurred. I sensed that the bear was talking with me and responding to my comments. He even seemed to smile. Yes, part of me was still scared, but not paralyzed or mentally frozen. I paid attention, felt all my emotions fully, and actually enjoyed the experience. Then the bear started to move in my direction, and I wasn't quite ready to hold out my hand to pet him. Before he got to me, he turned around and shuffled away. As I watched him meander off into the forest, I reflected on my extraordinary experience, one in which I learned that courage is inside of us all just waiting to rear its beautiful head.

We strengthen and develop our courage by using it. Don't let it go to waste. Trust in who you are and be all you were created to be by living a courageous life.

To have peace and confidence within our souls—
these are the beliefs that make for happiness.

~MAURICE MAETERLINCK

Have I not commanded you? Be strong and courageous.
Do not be frightened, and do not be dismayed, for
the Lord your God is with you wherever you go.

~JOSHUA 1:9

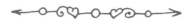

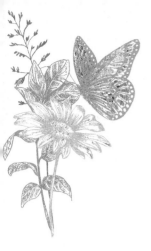

Chapter 12

Embracing Silence & Solitude to Enhance Each Day

May the Lord silence all flattering lips
and every boastful tongue.

~PSALM 12:3

Well-timed silence hath more eloquence than speech.

~MARTIN FARQUHAR TUPPER

*N*oise seems to be part of our everyday lives—from the alarm clock in the morning, to the traffic outside, to the never-ending sounds of voices, radio, television, smart phones and tablets. Our bodies and minds appear to acclimate to these outside intrusions. Or do they?

Over two decades ago, the Committee on Environmental Quality of the Federal Council for Science and Technology found that "growing numbers of researchers fear the dangerous and hazardous effects of intense noise on human health are seriously underestimated." Similarly, the late Vice President Nelson Rockefeller, when writing about the environmental crisis of our time, noted that when people are fully aware of the damage noise can inflict on man, "Peace and quiet will surely rank along with clean skies and pure waters as top priorities for our generation."

More recent studies suggest that we pay a price for adapting to noise: higher blood pressure, heart rate, and adrenaline secretion; heightened aggression; impaired resistance to disease; a sense of helplessness.

Studies indicate that when we can control noise, its effects are much less damaging.

I haven't been able to find many studies on the effects of quiet in repairing the stress of noise, but I know intuitively that most of us love quiet and need it desperately. Even when I go to see a movie in a theater, I wear earplugs to help turn down the volume of the soundtrack, which is much higher in decibels than my ears appreciate. We are so used to noise in our lives that silence can sometimes feel awkward and unsettling. On vacation, for instance, when quiet prevails, we may have trouble sleeping. But choosing times of silence can enrich the quality of our lives tremendously. If you find yourself overworked, stressed out, irritated, or tense, rather than heading for a coffee or snack break, maybe all you need is a silence break.

Everyone at some time has experienced the feeling of being overwhelmed by life. Everyone, too, has felt the need to escape, to find a quiet, secluded place to experience the peace of Spirit, the tranquility of God, to be alone with quiet thoughts. Creating times of silence in our life takes commitment and discipline. Most of the time, periods of silence must be scheduled into your day's activities or you'll never have any.

Maybe you can carve out times of silence while at home where you can be without radio, television, telephones, or voices. If you live in a family, maybe the best quiet time for you is early in the morning before others arise. In that silence, you can become more aware, more sensitive to your surroundings, and feel more in touch with the wholeness of life.

From quiet time or silence, you recognize the importance of solitude. Silence and solitude go hand in hand. In silence and solitude, you reconnect with the loving presence of God within you and all around you. Solitude helps to clear your channels, fosters peace, and brings spiritual lucidity. When you retreat from the outside world to go within, you can be at the very center of your being and reacquaint yourself with your spiritual nature—the essence of your being and all life.

Outside noise tends to drown out the inner life—the music of the soul. Only in silence and solitude can we go within and nurture our spiritual lives. Within each of us there is a silence waiting to be embraced. It's the harbor of the heart. When you rediscover that harbor, your life will never be the same. In the Bible we read, "There is silence in heaven" (**Revelations 8:1**). "For God alone my soul waits in silence." (**Psalm 62:1**).

Mystics, saints, and spiritual leaders have all advocated periods of silence and solitude for spiritual growth. St. John of the Cross writes that only in silence can the soul hear the Divine. Jesus prayed much by Himself and spent long hours in silent communion with God. Gandhi devoted every Monday to a day of silence. In silence he was better able to meditate and pray, to seek within himself the solutions to all the problems and responsibilities he carried. When I read about Gandhi's practice of silence and solitude several years ago, I was so inspired and moved that I decided to adopt a similar discipline in my life. So now one-half to one day a week and for two to three consecutive days with each change of season, I spend time in solitude, silence, prayer, and quiet. For this weekly respite from the world, it might be my long hike in the mountains alone. Even now, during this writing process, I'm choosing to spend as much time as possible in silence.

How do you feel about being alone? Aloneness is quite different from loneliness. This idea is expressed beautifully by Paul Tillich in *Courage to Be:*

> Our language has wisely sensed the two sides of being alone. It has created the word loneliness to express the pain of being alone. And it has created the word solitude to express the glory of being alone.

Loneliness is something you do to yourself. Have you ever experienced feeling lonely even when you're with other people? We're so used to being with others and so unaccustomed to being by ourselves that we've, in a sense, become a people and not person. We must reclaim ourselves and reconnect with our wholeness and the peace of solitude. Choose to make solitude your friend.

Even if you're married, you need times of privacy and solitude. In my counseling, I always encourage couples to spend occasional time alone, not only daily, but also at regular intervals during the week, month, and year. In this way, you regain your identity as individuals. You bring so much more to the marriage when you come from feeling whole, complete, and strong. Solitude fosters these qualities.

With a little creativity, a marriage can accommodate solitude and privacy. I have witnessed all types of arrangements, including separate vacations, private rooms in the house, living separately during the week and coming together on weekends, and having special times during the day in which each person is left alone.

I know several people who do everything possible to preclude being alone. Often this is because they have never tried it, they are afraid of loneliness, or are simply uncomfortable with themselves. They haven't yet discovered the peace of their own company. It's not scary to be by yourself; it's absolutely wonderful. Loneliness is not a state of being; it's simply a state of mind. You can choose to change your state of mind.

I realize that I live my life differently from most. I go to great lengths to secure my time of solitude and privacy. It's a great comfort to me to be by myself; it's like returning home to an old friend or lover after being away too long. Solitude is not a luxury. It is a right and a necessity.

Through the years I have gone on several vision quests. A vision quest is a time of solitude during which an individual can take time for looking into the soul, finding a new direction or path, or simply reconnecting with one's Higher Self, the part of you that's connected to God and Jesus. On these occasions, I usually go to the ocean or the mountains for a time of prayer, meditation, reflection, and aloneness. I spend much of my time outdoors, being open to the beauty and love all around me. In this peaceful, reflective time, the earth, the sky, the wind, the animals, the incredible beauty, and Divine Order of everything takes on a new and personal meaning. I commune with the trees, the moon, the stars lighting up the night sky, the flowers, and the animals. During this time, I choose to take a technology fast and take a break from television, radio, cell phone, internet, or other distractions that would take me away from my communion with God. Too much mental multitasking with technology can enervate our body and mind and cause us to lose perspective on living fully. It's okay to unplug now and then, and press the "reset" button! My vision quests always show me that the most profound lessons in life come to us through nature, solitude, and silence.

It is my contention that all the other good things we endeavor to provide for ourselves, including sound nutrition, daily exercise, and material wealth, will be of reduced value unless we learn to live in harmony with ourselves, which means knowing ourselves and finding peace in our own company. This peace is a natural occurrence of spending time alone in silence. In spending time alone we realize that we are never really alone and that we can live more fully by focusing on inner guidance rather than on externalities.

Embrace solitude. Walk in silence among the trees, in the mountains, by the ocean, with the sun and moon as your friends. Be by yourself, and experience a whole new way of celebrating yourself and life. Feel the heartbeat of silence. Bathe in its light and love. Know within yourself that you are a child of God, made in His image and likeness, and in your silence is Heaven.

It is better to keep your mouth closed and let people think
you are a fool than to open it and remove all doubt.
~Mark Twain

Each day find a few moments to walk in silence, still
your voice, and connect with the Lord Jesus who lives
inside the heart of those who have given their lives to
Him. Let go of excessive raucous activities in daily life.
Too much noise and chatter can ruin our inner antennae
that connects us to God. We must become ever watchful
for God's footsteps to come into our body temples.
~David Craddock

Chapter 13

Seeing the World through Sparkling Clear Eyes

*You can't depend on your eyes
when your imagination is out of focus.*

~MARK TWAIN

*Could a greater miracle take place than for us to
look through each other's eyes for an instant.*

~HENRY DAVID THOREAU

$\mathcal{M}$y wonderful mother, June, used to say the following to me: "Sometimes the eyes can say more than the mouth." How true that is! When you smile from the heart, your eyes sparkle and, as the saying goes, the eyes are the windows to the soul.

Through the yearlong process of writing this book, it was uncanny to me how many people with whom I came in contact around the country and world were having issues with their eyes and asked me for guidance on how to improve their vision. More than any other eye issue, many of my friends and clients were dealing with cataracts, which blur vision and can make it difficult to live a normal life. In fact, I met a few people who were diagnosed with cataracts in one or both eyes and were so afraid to have the cataract removal surgery that they opted, instead, to downgrade their lives and live more housebound because they couldn't drive anymore. With the advancements in cataract surgery, and with it usually being covered by insurance, I always suggest to others to go for the surgery so you can see clearly again.

Here's one of the many secrets to success: "Teach what you know." And as providence would have it, I learned in 2019 that I, too, had cataracts, so I made it my mission to learn everything I could about what causes them, how to prevent them, and the entire process of having them removed through eye surgery.

So in this chapter, if you are dealing with cataracts or know anyone who needs the cataract removal surgery, I will share my entire experience of having them removed and the glory of being able to see clearly again. There's no reason to be afraid of having cataracts removed if you have an outstanding ophthalmologist with a strong track record of performing these surgeries. So here's my story to, hopefully, give you guidance, let you know what to discuss with your own doctor, and to support you on your journey to see our beautiful world with greater focus and clarity.

He who can no longer pause to wonder and stand rapt
in awe, is as good as dead; his eyes are closed.

~ALBERT EINSTEIN

There was a knock at my front door and when I opened it, I saw tears in my neighbor's eyes and I thought, *What could possibly cause her to be so sad?* I invited her inside and we sat down at my kitchen table for a cup of hot tea together. Gloria had been away on a three-month business trip and noticed during the trip that her vision seemed to be getting cloudier. She described it as though she was looking through a dusty glass. So she decided to see an eye doctor for an exam the day before she traveled home. "He told me I have cataracts in both of my eyes and he recommended removing the cataracts with eye surgery," she said to me with trepidation. Gloria went on to say that she always had very sensitive eyes and the thought of a doctor going inside her eyes during surgery to remove each lens and replace it with a new lens was daunting to her and she was afraid to even move forward.

*It opens the lungs, washes the countenance, exercises
the eyes, and softens down the temper, so cry away.*

~CHARLES DICKENS

Gloria is not alone. As mentioned above, I've known people who have been diagnosed with cataracts and feel quite reluctant to have surgery. She asked me to recommend the best ophthalmologist (a medical doctor who treats disorders and diseases of the eye) in the Southern California area with whom she could consult and have a second opinion. "Maybe the doctor I saw last week on the East Coast was wrong and I don't really have cataracts, and all I need is to reduce my stress and get extra sleep to correct my increasingly blurry vision."

Choosing the Best Eye Doctor

What Gloria was about to find out from me was that while she was away, I was diagnosed with cataracts in both of my eyes and already had them removed. My doctor of choice, because he's the best, is Brian Boxer Wachler, MD, in Beverly Hills, and I have been going to him for decades for my annual eye checkups and more.

I told Gloria that Dr. Brian is regarded as one of the very top leaders in the world in the field of vision correction. In fact, Dr. Brian is the "Surgeon's Surgeon" since so many other doctors and surgeons go to Dr. Brian for surgery on their own eyes. And it's not just people and doctors from Southern California who call him their doctor. Over the years and decades, I have met many people in his waiting room area during my countless visits who have traveled from different states and countries to see Dr. Brian and have him do their eye surgeries. That's how I feel about him, too. He's the eye doctor who has my total trust and I know many people who are his patients and also feel the same way. If you need eye surgery, make sure you go to an excellent ophthalmologist.

Not only is Dr. Brian an expert in eye disorders and surgery, but he is also a genuinely kind, thoughtful, and down-to-earth person with the best bedside manner I've ever experienced in any doctor's office. I never feel rushed; he answers all of my questions; he actually looks at you when you are speaking to him rather than writing notes and looking at the paperwork—which so many other doctors do these days; and he has a great sense of humor. He instills confidence in his patients and the knowledge we need to make the best decisions for our eyes. In fact, he is so personable and brilliant in his surgical work that he is a frequent guest on television talk shows like *The Doctors, The Today Show, Good Morning America, Ellen, CNN,* and many more. And it's not just other surgeons and doctors and everyday folks that see him. He is the surgeon for countless world-class athletes, TV and movie celebrities, Fortune 500 Presidents and CEOs, and others who, like myself, want the best and most capable doctor to work on our eyes.

So for the next 30 minutes with Gloria while sipping our tea, I described in detail my very positive experience with getting my cataracts removed. And this is what I told her, in case you or someone you know will find this information helpful.

You need at least two weeks between the two cataract removal surgeries if you have one in each eye. It can be more time, but not less than two weeks. I told Gloria how my vision was slowly getting more dulled over the months and getting stronger readers wasn't helping me. I thought it had to do with too much time sitting in front of my computer screen, which, by the way, is not good for our eyes. I, too, was concerned and went to Dr. Brian, who diagnosed me with cataracts in both of my eyes.

What Causes Cataracts to Develop?

Cataracts can develop from normal aging, from an eye injury, certain medications, or genetic congenital defect. Risk factors include diabetes, smoking, prolonged exposure to sunlight, and alcohol. Prevention includes wearing sunglasses and avoiding smoking. When you have cataracts, it may cause blurred and dulled vision, sensitivity to light, and glare and/or ghost images. What happened with me is that the cataracts changed my vision enough that it interfered with the quality in my daily life, mostly likely due to too much computer screen time combined with too much Southern California sunlight without always wearing sunglasses. So I opted to have them removed as soon as I found out the diagnosis from Dr. Brian. There really is no other option. Surgery is the only way to remove a cataract. Yes, you could opt to forgo surgery and continue to wear glasses, but the quality of vision with a clouded lens can be diminished. A few people I know, as referred to earlier, are unable to drive anymore and are essentially prisoners in their home (unless they use rideshare or have neighbors help them out) because they have cataracts in each of their eyes and are afraid to have cataract removal surgery. Yes, of course, I will be sharing this book's chapter with them and encouraging them to schedule appointments with Dr. Brian or find another excellent ophthalmologist.

Keep your eyes on the stars, and your feet on the ground.
~Theodore Roosevelt

The course of action would probably be similar for you in what I am describing here. My cataract surgery was done at a specialty surgical center in Beverly Hills near Dr. Brian's office. Both of my surgeries were completely painless, easy, and fast. Yes, I was a little nervous for the first one, not knowing exactly what it would be like, and it was only because of my full confidence in Dr. Brian that I wasn't racked on the first surgery day. Then, for the second cataract removal surgery two weeks later, knowing already about the proven, painless, efficacious process, I actually looked forward, with alacrity, to the surgery.

How Is Cataract Surgery Performed and What Artificial Lens to Choose?

I learned from Dr. Brian that cataract surgery removal starts with a capsulotomy, which refers to creating an opening around the capsule that holds the lens (cataract). Next, an ultrasound instrument is used to break down and remove the cataract. Once the lens is removed, an artificial lens (IOL = intraocular lens) is inserted. Prior to the surgery day for each eye, Dr. Brian discussed with me the IOL options and which would be best for me. It's based on whether you are treating nearsightedness/myopia, farsightedness/hyperopia, and astigmatism. Some newer IOLs referred to as multifocal or accommodating IOLs can provide near, intermediate (computer distance), and distance vision, and this one, Dr. Brian and I decided together, was best to insert in my left eye. For the right eye, we opted for a monovision IOL and it worked well for my eye issues.

> *The hardest thing to see is what is in front of your eyes.*
> ~JOHANN WOLFGANG VON GOETHE

The Day of Surgery: What to Expect

At the surgical center, I was attended to with multiple visits by nurses and the anesthesiologist to go over my chart and particulars, administer eye drops, and answer any questions. Their adeptness took away much of my anxiety. And, by the way, I had no anxiety whatsoever for the second cataract removal surgery because I knew how painless and successful it would be. Dr. Brian visited me before the surgery, gave me a few instructions during the surgery on moving my eye in different directions, and then followed up with me when I was in recovery. He also called me the evening after each surgery, as he does with all of his surgery patients, to see how I was doing. The surgeries were only about 15 minutes for each eye, and I can say, in all honesty, that there was absolutely no pain. I could feel a little pressure in the eyes during surgery, but there was no pain because they use very effective numbing drops. You must have someone you know drive you to and from the surgical center. When I arrived home after surgery, I rested for the rest of the day, and still without any pain at all.

In addition to the numbing drops, the anesthesiologist administers an anesthetic technique where a mild dose of sedation is applied to induce anxiolysis (anxiety relief). In other words, as the patient, I was not unconscious, but simply lightly sedated. It's often referred to as a "twilight state," where a patient is relaxed and "sleepy," able to follow simple directions by the doctor, and is still responsive. It's designed to make the patient feel more comfortable, and it was quite effective, indeed, for me.

Eyes that do not cry, do not see.

~Swedish Proverb

After My Cataract Removal Surgeries

After cataract removal surgery, part of the process is returning to his office the day after, and also a week later for two follow-up, post-op appointments. After the first surgery on my left eye, I no longer needed to use my readers with the insertion of the multifocal lens, which I had been wearing for only very small print for years. Of course, the vision in my right eye was still cloudy and the second surgery date could not arrive soon enough for me. So for only two weeks, I experienced a period of imbalance between the two eyes (anisometropia), and this usually cannot be corrected with glasses because of the marked difference in the prescriptions. I was given a variety of eye drops that I needed to bring with me to the surgery center where the nurses covered in detail how to use them—one for only a week and the others for three to six weeks following surgery. It was simple to adhere to this eye drop routine.

Within three days of the second surgery, my overall vision was better than it's been for years and continued to get even better over the following weeks after both surgeries. It was a miracle to me that a surgical procedure that took about 15 minutes for each eye and was pain-free could result in such positive results.

As I was telling Gloria about my very positive experience with cataract removal surgery, I could see her entire demeanor change before my eyes from stressed out and sad to hopeful and happy, as I always knew her to be. Before she even left my home, Gloria used my telephone to ring up Dr. Brian's office and schedule an appointment for an eye exam. I'm happy to report that her results with two cataract surgeries were as positive as mine, and she can now see superbly without readers, too. Not long ago, she said to me, "I am feeling decades younger since my cataract removal surgeries and my vision is now sharp and refreshed."

When I look into the future, it's so bright it burns my eyes.

~Oprah Winfrey

Nutritional Eye Supplements

Dr. Brian offers his patients and others his supplement called Optimal Flax, which is pure, organic, cold-pressed flaxseed oil. He recommends taking 3,000 mg a day for six months after surgery. Flaxseed oil is a natural anti-inflammatory, rich in omega-3s, and has many health benefits, including heart and brain health. The reason Dr. Brian recommends this after surgery is to increase the tear film quality, producing more natural tears. This is because eyes can feel dry after surgery, sometimes feeling a foreign body sensation in the eyes, like an eyelash in the eye.

While I take his supplement, I also grind up organic, golden flaxseed once a week (about one cup max so it's always fresh each week), put it in a closed container in the refrigerator, and have about 2 tablespoons a day either sprinkled on my salads or other dishes, or stirred into water or juice. The nutty, delicious taste of the freshly ground flaxseed makes it so enjoyable and welcoming to incorporate in my daily diet. Grind it yourself in a small grinder you can get for a low cost—like a coffee grinder. However, I would keep it dedicated to seeds and nuts and if you also grind coffee beans, then have a second grinder dedicated just for your beans so the flavors don't marry. I also use this small device for grinding other seeds and nuts. It's one of the many angel gadgets I have in my kitchen and wouldn't be without. In Chapter 17, you will see that I've also recommended whole flaxseed in your smoothies as a thickener and also to give any smoothie a nutritional boost. The blender grinds them up so that they are digestible; otherwise, they will go right through you and look back up at you from the toilet bowl 🙂.

In addition to flaxseed, I encourage you to take a comprehensive, high-quality nutritional supplement to use long-term to help support healthy eye function, including macular health. Look for these ingredients when finding the best supplement to take to support ocular and macular health: beta-carotene, vitamin C, vitamin E, zinc, copper, lutein, bilberry, eyebright, bioflavonoids, astaxanthin, zeaxanthin, and CoQ10. (I get most of my eye and other nutritional supplements and Olbas products at PennHerb.com.)

You should still wear sunglasses when outdoors to help slow the natural aging of the eyes. Sunglasses should always have thick enough sides so that the sunlight is blocked out and make sure your eyes are protected from UVA light in your car.

> *"The eye is the lamp of the body. If your eyes are healthy,*
> *your whole body will be full of light."*
>
> ~MATTHEW 6:22

UVA Light in Your Car's Side Window Can Lead to Cataracts

Wondering why there were more cataract issues in people's left eyes, along with skin cancers on the left side of the face, Dr. Brian conducted a study that was published in 2016 in *JAMA Ophthalmology*. The objective was to assess the level of UVA light protection in the front windshields and side windows of automobiles. In this cross-sectional study, 29 automobiles from 15 automobile manufacturers were analyzed. The outside ambient UVA radiation, along with UVA radiation behind the front windshield and behind the driver's side window of all automobiles, was measured. The years of the automobiles ranged from 1990 to 2014, with an average year of 2010. The automobile dealerships were located in Los Angeles, CA.

In this study, measurements were taken in the amount of UVA blockage from windshields and side windows. The average percentage of the front-windshield UVA blockage was 96% and was higher than the average percentage of side-window blockage, which was 71%. A high level of side-window UVA blockage (>90%) was found in only 4 of 29 automobiles (13.8%).

Here were his conclusions and relevance: "The level of front-windshield UVA protection was consistently high among automobiles. The level of side-window UVA protection was lower and highly variable. These results may, in part, explain the reported increased rates of cataracts in the left eyes and left-sided facial skin cancer. Automakers may wish to consider increasing the degree of UVA protection in the side windows of automobiles." I wholeheartedly agree!

Dr. Brian's patients can request UV cards to be mailed to them to test their car windows. If your UVA levels are high, you can go to a window-tinting company and have a clear, UV film placed on the side windows. This is exactly what I did on my car to both the driver and passenger sides.

If you wish to make an appointment with Dr. Brian, please call his office at 310-860-1900 or 888-982-1900. I also encourage you to visit his informative website: BoxerWachler.com. If you can't get to see Dr. Brian, carefully research ophthalmologists and get referrals to find the best doctor in your state.

The face is the mirror of the mind, and eyes without speaking confess the secrets of the heart.

~St. Jerome

For beautiful eyes, look for the good in others; for beautiful lips, speak only words of kindness; and for poise, walk in the knowledge that you are never alone.

~Audrey Hepburn

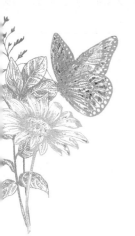

Intermission

Humor Time, Part 2

THE BUTTERFLY & STUD

Mr. and Mrs. Adams met their demise in a common accident and proceeded to Heaven together. St. Peter met them at the pearly gates and told them they had arrived at a very fortunate time, as it was Bargain Day and they would be allowed to return to earth for 48 hours and do or be anything they wanted.

"Really?" exclaimed Mrs. Adams. "Can we really be anything we want?"

"Absolutely," answered St. Peter. "Just name it and your wish will be granted."

"Oh, St. Peter," said Mrs. Adams, "all my life I've wanted to be a butterfly. May I really be a butterfly for 48 hours?"

"Certainly," said St. Peter. "Go and have a wonderful time," and off she went.

Then Mr. Adams said, "St. Peter, all my life I've wanted to be a stud. May I really be a stud for 48 hours?"

"You may, indeed," answered St. Peter. "Go, and enjoy!"

A little before the 48-hour period ended, Mrs. Adams returned and said to St. Peter, "I had a perfectly delightful day. I visited one orchard after another, smelled the roses and flowers blooming in the gardens, and even tasted honey from a honeysuckle. It was lovely and I had a fabulous time. Thank you so much, St. Peter, I'll never forget it."

"Welcome to heaven," St. Peter replied. And Mrs. Adams proceeded through the pearly gates.

A little while later she returned and asked, "St. Peter, where is my husband? I've looked all over Heaven and I can't find him. Do you know where he is?"

"Well," answered St. Peter, "the last time I saw him he was on a tire headed for Colorado!"

(Watch out for what you ask for. You just might get it!)

MINISTER, SEX & SAILING

A minister was asked to speak before a young lady's health symposium. When his wife asked him what he intended to talk about, he was too embarrassed to tell her he had been asked to talk about sex, so he told her he was going to talk about sailing.

"Oh, that's nice, dear," she said.

The morning after the lecture, a young lady who had attended the symposium recognized the minister's wife in the grocery store and said to her, "Your husband gave a marvelous talk last night. He certainly has a unique perspective on the subject."

"That's odd," replied the wife. "He's only done it twice. The first time he threw up and the second time, his hat blew off!"

HAPPY HUNTING

A housewife heard a knock at her front door and opened it to find two small boys. One was holding a list.

"Lady," he said, "me and my brother are on a treasure hunt. Do you have three grains of wheat, a pork chop bone, or a used piece of carbon paper?"

"I don't have any of those things," the woman responded. "That's a very hard list. What kind of treasure hunt is this?"

"If we find everything on this list," said the boy, "we win a dollar!"

"And who's going to give you the dollar," asked the woman.

The boy answered, "Our babysitter's boyfriend!"

BROCCOLI & THE MARKET

Early Monday morning a woman goes to the market to get some broccoli. Just after the produce was all neatly arranged, she forages through the offerings, moving everything around, trying to locate broccoli. The produce manager comes over and says, "Lady, we don't have any broccoli now. Please stop messing up the produce."

Early the following Monday, she goes back and again starts dishelving everything. And again the produce manager tells her there's no broccoli—it's out of season.

Finally, the next week she's back again, and before she starts to mess everything up, the manager says to her:

"Lady, is there a *ba* in banana?"

Yes, there's a ba in banana.

"Is there a *cab* in cabbage?"

Yes, there's a cab in cabbage.

"Well, is there a *fig* in broccoli?"

No, there's no fig in broccoli.

"That's what I've been trying to tell you!"

LIGHT LEAKING

I once knew a man who climbed up to a mountaintop and reached up to God. He stretched his arms to heaven and cried, "Fill me full of Light! I'm ready. I'm waiting!"

The voice of God answered him and said: "I'm always filling you with Light—but you keep leaking."

BOY THINKS "THE KING" IS ELVIS

There's a story about a little boy who went with his family to his church during Christmastime to see a concert featuring a live nativity scene. The little boy was not paying much attention.

As the wise men began marching down the center aisle toward the manger, his dad leaned over and whispered to his son, "Look, Johnny, you're missing it! Here comes the King!"

Johnny jumped up, looked over the balcony railing, and asked, "That's Elvis?!"

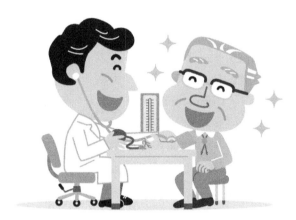

HEALTHY 75-YEAR-OLD

A healthy, robust, vibrant 75-year-old man went to see his doctor for his annual physical. The doctor, in seeing how healthy he was, just had to ask him how his father died. The man replied, "What do you mean, my father is still living, he's 100 years old and in great health."

Then the doctor just had to ask how his grandfather died. And once again, the man replied, "My grandfather is still living too. He's 125 and also in great health. In fact, next week he's getting married."

To that the doctor quipped, "Why would he want to do something like that?"

And the man blurted back, "Who says he wants to."

FLY LIKE AN EAGLE–INSPIRATION

A little Native American boy was out playing in the woods and he found an egg that had fallen out of its nest. So he took it home as a keepsake. When he showed it to his father, he told his son to take it back because it was an eagle's egg.

But he disobeyed his father and kept it instead. He hid it in the chicken coop. Shortly thereafter it hatched and acted like it was a chicken. It pecked and scratched and ran around in the dirt like all the other chickens. (*We humans often mimic the behavior and beliefs of others around us.*)

One day a great eagle flew overhead. And the little chick eagle looked up and saw this majestic eagle in all its glory flying overhead. Well, this little chick eagle was inspired and wanted to be just like that eagle in the sky. (*The potential is always within you.*)

So little chick eagle told all his fellow chick buddies, "I'm going to be like that eagle one day. I'll soar in the clouds." They all laughed at him and he began to doubt his dreams

He didn't know his true self, didn't believe in his heart—but instead made what others were saying much more important and he lived his life as a chicken and died that way.

The more we listen to other people rather than to what our heart is telling us and what God is whispering to us, we limit our ability to soar—to fly. Choose to live a God-centered life and you will take flight.

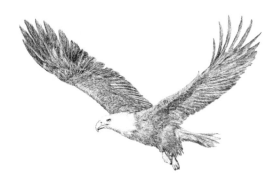

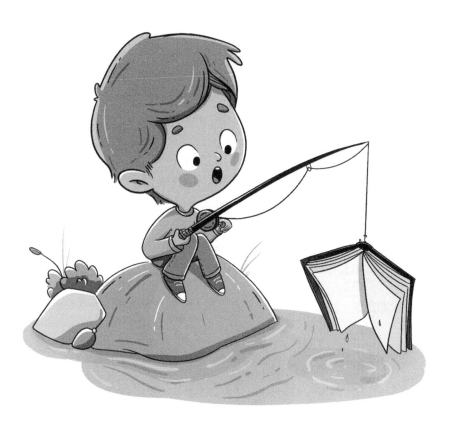

Part 5

16 Simple Ways to Enrich the Quality of Your Life

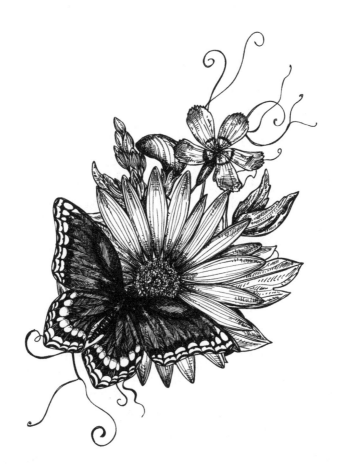

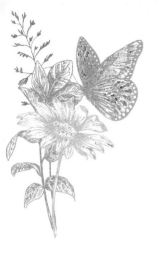

Chapter 14

Filling Your Rewarding Life with Vim & Verve

Everyone is born a genius,
but the process of living de-geniuses them.

~Buckminster Fuller

It is not that I am so smart. But I stay with the questions longer.

~Albert Einstein

$\mathcal{E}$ach of us faces tremendous challenges every day. As we get up each morning, we may face myriad stressors—getting the kids off to school, driving in bumper-to-bumper traffic, presenting a career-making (or career-breaking) report to the boss, balancing the household budget, and so much more. It can seem like there is not enough time in the day to accomplish all you need to do. These are just some of the ways everyday life can get us down. If poorly managed, these challenges can lead to many forms of stress, depression, and anxiety.

Stress is a fact of life, but you can choose not to make it a way of life for you. By incorporating some or most of the tips below, you will experience more joy and less stress. You will be well on your way to creating a healthy, happy, peaceful, fulfilling, and soul-satisfying life. Not only do these tips help assuage stress, they also help prevent and alleviate disease and depression, boost energy, and restore youthful vitality.

Living a stress-free life is not a reasonable goal. The real goal is to learn to deal with stress actively and effectively. Although that's easier for some people than others, studies suggest that anyone can learn to cope better. But I don't want you to just cope; I want you to *thrive*—to be vibrantly healthy, joyful, and balanced. Your path is always being lit by God's Light, and you are always being guided in the direction of your dreams. Open up to this guidance by affirming—"I AM . . . divinely guided and inspired."

Thy word is a lamp unto my feet,
and a light unto my path.

~PSALM 119:105

Here are 16 simple, yet essential, choices that I recommend and use with clients, friends, and family members to bring more vitality and purpose into your body and life. While I have covered much of this information throughout the book in various chapters, here it is for quick reference all in one chapter. I have found these tips to be profoundly efficacious and practicable. Making a new life for yourself is simply a matter of choice. So today, *choose to . . .*

1. Sleep your way to youthful vitality.

There is nothing more restorative for your body than a good night's sleep, night after night after night. Consistent lack of sleep can lead to a variety of health problems, including toxic buildup, weight gain, accelerated aging, depression, irritability and impatience, low sex drive, memory loss, lethargy, relationship problems, accidents, and at least 1,500 reported "drowsy driving" fatalities each year. Studies reveal that *driving on only 6 hours of sleep is like driving drunk.* Cars are so cozy and comfortable these days, and cruise control doesn't help. The instant you feel drowsy at the wheel of an automobile—when your eyelids get heavy—get off the road!

People are sleeping less now than they did a century ago, thanks to electric lighting and the shift to an urban, industrialized economy, not to mention late-night television and cellphone or tablet activity. The result is a disruption of basic body metabolism. With workloads and daily stress increasing for many of us, sleep issues loom larger than ever. Let's take a brief look at sleep and how lack of it affects us as individuals and as a society.

At the University of Chicago, Karine Spiegel and colleagues asked research participants to stay in bed just 4 hours per night for six nights, then 12 hours per night for the next seven nights. When subjects were sleep deprived, their blood sugars, cortisol, and sympathetic nervous system activity rose, and thyrotropin, which regulates thyroid function, fell. In other words, the results of this study show that chronic sleep deprivation forces the body into a fight-or-flight response, pushing blood sugars and other hormone-related functions out of kilter.

Higher cortisol levels, among other things, lead to memory loss, an increase in fat storage, and a decrease in muscle—the perfect combination if you want to lower metabolism and gain weight easily. But if you want to increase muscle mass, which is necessary to create a fit, lean, healthy body, you need at least 8 hours of sound sleep nightly to encourage muscle maintenance and growth and the release of the human growth hormone, which helps keep you youthful and strong. Put another way, *sleeping more can make you slimmer.*

Sleep deprivation also may accelerate the aging process. In the same Spiegel study, participants who only slept 4 hours per night for one week metabolized glucose 40% more slowly than usual, which is similar to the rate seen in elderly people. Glucose metabolism quickly returned to normal after participants got a full night's sleep every night for a week.

So how do you know if you are sleep deprived? World-renowned sleep expert Dr. William C. Dement, author of *The Promise of Sleep*, says that if you become sluggish, drowsy, or fatigued, particularly after lunch or in the middle of the afternoon, you are sleep deprived. If you have difficulty getting up in the morning—one of my clients often sleeps through two alarms—you're sleep deprived.

Ninety-five percent of Americans suffer from a sleep disorder at some time in their lives, and 60% suffer from some persistent sleep disorder, according to Dement's research. When it comes to sleep, he says, "Most people require a minimum of eight hours nightly." Every hour you lose adds to your sleep indebtedness, and you cannot expect to catch up by sleeping late one day a week. The lost sleep accumulates progressively and contributes to long-term health problems. And this doesn't just pertain to adults. Children and teens actually need even more sleep than adults. Sleep loss affects how they learn, causes accidents, increases the likelihood of depression, and can lead to violent or aggressive behavior.

Recognizing that many of us simply can't get to bed any earlier or get up any later, Dement recommends napping. A few enlightened businesses are adopting the pioneering view that napping actually can promote productivity. Some companies even provide special nap rooms for employees. Naps should be recognized as a powerful tool in battling fatigue. However, if you have insomnia, naps can actually aggravate your night's sleep. By taking the edge off your sleepiness, an afternoon nap may make it even harder for you to sleep at night. In other words, if you are sleepy because of insomnia, napping should be *avoided*.

Naps are also *not* recommended after meals. It's natural to want to nap after eating because distension of the stomach from the meal increases the deep-sleep drive. The problem is that if you overeat, the digestive process may interfere with the *quality* of your sleep, and conversely, sleep may interfere with the digestive process. You are better off to allow digestion to occur *before* sleeping, since both digestion and sleep tend to work better when performed separately.

Here are five tips for better sleep:

❖ **MORNING EXERCISE HELPS YOU SLEEP AT NIGHT.** If you're not a morning person, exercise at least four hours before bedtime—any closer and you'll be too revved up.

❖ **INCREASE EVENING BODY HEAT FOR DEEPER SLEEP.** A hot bath, sauna, or Jacuzzi two hours before bedtime increases melatonin as the body temperature drops after the heat therapy is over. This overall increased body temperature, with its accompanying big drop back to normal, helps promote sound, deep sleep.

❖ **MAKE SURE THE BED IS FOR SLEEP AND SEX ONLY.** Avoid working, eating, or watching TV in bed. Reading until you fall asleep is okay, but try to read inspirational, uplifting, or calming books such as *Relentless* by John Tesh or my book *Be the Change* ☺.

❖ **CREATE A CONDUCIVE ENVIRONMENT.** Sleep in natural fiber pajamas in a dark and quiet room, with fresh air and green plants. A cool room and cool pillow are also helpful. Two or three drops of pure essential lavender oil on your pillow promotes relaxation and calm. And, of course, a good mattress and a few pillows are essential.

❖ **DON'T EAT OR DRINK LIQUIDS TOO CLOSE TO BEDTIME.** Choose your evening meals wisely. Large, spicy meals within 2 to 3 hours of bedtime undermine deep sleep. Alcohol is a stimulant and blocks the restful sleep experienced during the REM (rapid eye movement) cycle. While I advocate drinking several glasses of pure, alkaline water throughout the day, cut off your water intake within two hours of bedtime to cut down on nighttime bathroom visits and to take extra stress off your kidneys. Sweet dreams!

2. Hydrate your body with purified water.

Without water, life does not exist. Before scientists look for any form of life on other planets, they first look for any sign of water. Over 70% of our body weight is water; that's about 10 gallons of water for a 120-pound person. We're bundles of water wrapped in skin standing on two feet.

Water is a strong solvent that carries many invisible ingredients: minerals, oxygen, hydrogen, nutrients, waste products, pollutants, etc. Inside the human body, blood (90% of which is water) circulates throughout the body distributing nutrients and oxygen, and collecting wastes and carbon dioxide. Every substance deep in our body was brought there by blood ("the river of life") and can be carried out by blood. When a person loses 20 pounds of weight through a diet program, that 20 pounds of substance comes out of the body through urine, which is why any diet program requires drinking a lot of water.

Water is very important in helping to maintain a healthy metabolic rate. At least two quarts a day, between meals, is essential—more if you're physically very active or take an infrared sauna frequently, as I do. That's at least eight glasses of water daily. Freshly squeezed fruit or vegetable juices and natural teas without caffeine can count towards your water tally. But keep in mind that not all liquid is alike. While liquids are wet, some are actually *anti*water. Alcohol, sodas, coffee, and other caffeinated beverages act as diuretics, thus increasing your need for more water during the day.

We often turn to food when we're really just thirsty. Water makes you feel fuller and suppresses your appetite naturally. Have a large glass of water about 15 to 20 minutes before each meal or snack. If you are interested in losing some body fat, listen up. Simply drinking purified water—between 10 and 14 glasses of water a day, and not changing anything else—not food or exercise—helps with fat loss and reshaping the body.

Water makes you feel fuller and suppresses your appetite naturally.

The liver's main functions are detoxification and regulation of metabolism. The kidneys can get rid of toxins and spare the liver if they have sufficient water. This allows the liver to metabolize more fat. Adequate water also will decrease bloating and edema caused by fluid accumulation by flushing out sodium, acidic wastes, and other toxins. A high water intake also helps relieve constipation by keeping your stools soft. Your urine should be clear, light-colored, and plentiful. Drink even more water in hot weather, low humidity (such as desert environments or air traveling), high altitude, when you're ill or stressed, when you want to accelerate fat loss, or when you're pregnant.

The best water to drink, in my estimation, is purified water. A few drops of fresh lemon juice in water is my favorite way to drink it. It adds to the taste, increases the nutritional value, and assists in healing and detoxification. Lemon in hot water first thing in the morning is an excellent laxative. Make a habit of drinking water. As written in the discerning book, *Water The Ultimate Cure*, by Steve Meyerowitz, "According to a survey, the reason most people don't drink as much as they know they ought to, is lack of time or being too busy. Decide to drink water before every meal. Set objectives for yourself such as drinking before you leave the house, and first thing upon your return, or before you start work. Take water breaks instead of coffee breaks." He also recommends, as I do, drinking one-half ounce daily for every pound you weigh. Thus, a 150-pound person drinks 75 ounces, or approximately 2.5 quarts. Here's my general rule of thumb: Drink one glass every hour so that your urine comes out clear, not dark yellow.

3. Alkalize and energize.

In his popular book, *Alkalize or Die*, author and friend Dr. Theodore A. Baroody writes about the importance of living a lifestyle that supports alkalinity. When foods are eaten, they are broken down into small nutrients and delivered to each and every cell in the body. These nutrients are burned with oxygen in a slow, controlled manner to supply the necessary energy for us to function. After oxidation, these nutrients become waste products. Gourmet or junk food, *all* foods make waste products. The difference between healthful food and unhealthful food is the amount and kind of wastes produced: acid or alkaline. Human cells die in about four weeks: some regenerate and some are destroyed. Dead cells are waste products. All waste products need to be discarded from the body, mostly through urine and perspiration. Most of these wastes are acidic; therefore, when we excrete them, our urine is acidic and our skin is acidic.

Most of us overwork, stay up late, get up early, and stress ourselves to the limit without giving ourselves time to rest. Most people like to eat meat and refined grains and enjoy colas and other soft drinks, which are all highly acidic foods and drinks. Furthermore, the polluted environment kills our healthy cells, thus producing more acidic wastes. This means that we cannot get rid of 100% of the acidic wastes that we make daily, and these leftover wastes are stored somewhere within our bodies.

Since our blood and cellular fluids must be slightly alkaline to sustain life, the body converts liquid acidic wastes into solid wastes. Solidification of liquid acid wastes is the body's defense mechanism to survive. Some of these acid wastes include cholesterol, fatty acid, uric acid, kidney stones, phosphates, sulfates, urates, and gallstones, and they accumulate in many places throughout our body.

One of the biggest problems caused by the buildup of acidic wastes is the fact that *acid coagulates blood*. When blood becomes thicker, it clogs up the capillaries, which is why so many adult diseases require blood thinners as part of their treatment. It is commonly known that degenerative diseases are caused by poor blood circulation. Where there is an accumulation of acidic wastes, and the local capillaries are clogged, any organ(s) in that area will not be getting an adequate blood supply, eventually leading to dysfunction of that organ(s).

Doctors have found that more than 150 degenerative diseases are associated with acidity, including cancer, diabetes, arthritis, heart disease, and gallstones and kidney stones. All diseases thrive in an acidic, oxygen-poor environment.

The symbol "pH" (power of hydrogen) is a measurement of how acidic or alkaline a substance is. The pH scale goes from 1–14. For example, a reading of 1 pH would be acidic, a reading of 7 pH would be neutral, and a reading of 14 pH would be alkaline.

> Doctors have found that more than 150 degenerative diseases are associated with acidity . . .

Keep in mind that a drop in every point on the pH scale is 10 times more acid (i.e., from 7 to 6 is 10 times, from 7 to 5 is 100 times, etc.). From 7 to 2 is 100,000 times more acidic! And sodas are in the acidic range of 2 pH. Over the long term, the effects of sodas are devastating to the body. Acidity, sugars, and artificial sweeteners can shorten your life. In fact, *it takes 32 glasses of alkaline water at a pH of 9 to neutralize the acid from one 12-ounce cola or soda.* When you drink sodas, the body uses up reserves of its own stored alkaline buffers—mainly calcium from the bones and DNA—to raise the body's alkalinity levels, especially to maintain proper blood alkaline pH levels. Acidic blood levels can cause death!

If you want to know your current acid-alkaline balance, you can check your pH with a simple saliva test by using litmus paper that comes with a color chart. To properly check your saliva pH, bring up your saliva twice and spit it out. Bring it up a third time, but don't spit it out. Put the litmus strip under your tongue and wet it with your saliva. To find your pH level, match the color of the litmus strip to the corresponding color on the chart. Your goal is to have an alkaline (7.1–7.5) pH level. Note that it is natural for you to be more alkaline in the morning and more acidic at night.

Most of the degenerative diseases we call "old-age diseases," like memory loss, osteoporosis, arthritis, diabetes, and hypertension, are actually lifestyle diseases caused by acidosis, an overall poor diet (especially a lack of leafy green vegetables), improper digestion, and too much stress. (Refer to Chapter 18 for the best leafy greens.)

So how can you alkalize your body? Baroody suggests following an 80-20 dietary rule. Choose 80% percent alkaline-forming foods and drinks and 20% acid-forming foods and drinks for vibrant health. His best-selling book, *Alkalize or Die*, breaks down all the foods in categories of acid, alkaline, or neutral. In a nutshell, most fruits and vegetables are alkaline and most other foods, including meat, dairy, fish, fowl, grains, seeds, and nuts are acid-forming, with a few exceptions. He recommends as an optimum diet building up to eating 75% fresh and raw plant-based foods and 25% cooked foods. He encourages the daily practice of meditation, deep breathing, exercise, deep sleep, and positive thinking—all of which increase alkalinity.

I choose to eat a vegetable-centric, alkaline-rich diet and include daily fresh vegetable juices and/or green smoothies, and add to my meals a few whole grains (like brown rice, millet, or quinoa), fresh sprouts, some nuts and seeds (like walnuts, almonds, cashews, and sunflower seeds), carbohydrates (like sweet potatoes), legumes (such as lentils and black beans), nut milk (usually homemade from raw, organic almonds), and always lots of large leafy green salads (with oodles of raw vegetables in them). Often, the salad is my main meal in which I add sprouts, beans, nuts, raw homemade hummus, and more. I even make all kinds delicious, unheated, dairy-free nut "cheeses" and creamy sauces from cashews, sunflower seeds, almonds, oats, and more.

One of the quickest and best ways to improve health and increase alkalinity is to make fresh vegetable juice every day. Chlorophyll, which gives green vegetables their color, builds the blood and powerfully alkalizes the system. I'll cover the importance of juicing in an upcoming tip.

For over 20 years, I have used an **Ionizer Plus** water device in my kitchen to make fresh, purified, alkaline water. This salubrious product will make a positive difference in your body by increasing your alkalinity, immunity, and energy, and helping to rejuvenate your body and look younger. Please visit my website, SusanSmithJones.com and under "Favorite Products," you will find many articles on the benefits of this health-enhancing alkaline water machine, the **Ionizer Plus**, that I would not be without.

Another way to increase your body's alkalinity is through exposure to direct sunlight.

4. Embrace healthy doses of natural sunlight.

The sun is the source of light and warmth and sustains our existence. It provides the energy for plants to photosynthesize the products necessary for growth. This energy is then stored in plants in the form of carbohydrates, proteins, and fats, and is transferred to us upon consumption. In a sense, the cycle of life also can be called the cycle of light. Raw plant foods are so beneficial for us because we're taking life-giving sunlight into our bodies.

> . . . the best way to get optimal levels of this nutrient is through exposure to the ultraviolet (UV) rays of the sun . . .

But the sun also has been getting a lot of bad press lately, and while baking in the sun is clearly not good for us, the latest research shows that short bouts of exposure without sunblock may yield significant health benefits, from helping to prevent some cancers to warding off depression, increasing fitness and libido, and lowering cholesterol, blood sugar, and blood pressure. I recommend short bouts of direct sunlight to help produce proper hormonal levels and to assist alkaline-acid balances.

Vitamin D is a fat-soluble vitamin found in limited quantities in foods; however, for most people, the best way to get optimal levels of this nutrient is through exposure to the ultraviolet (UV) rays of the sun, which triggers vitamin D synthesis in the skin. A fat-soluble nutrient, Vitamin D can be stored in the body for use in periods of no sunshine.

For light-skinned people like myself, "10 to 15 minutes of sun exposure at least two times per week to the face, arms, hands, or back without sunscreen is usually sufficient to provide adequate vitamin D" (Dietary Supplement Fact Sheet: Vitamin D, NIH Clinical Center, p. 1). Dark-skinned people require up to six times that amount of exposure to arrive at the same level of vitamin D as fair-skinned people. This sunshine supplement helps prevent disease and is also needed for calcium absorption, and thus plays an important role in protecting against osteoporosis, bone fractures, and PMS. Scientific findings further indicate that vitamin D may affect mood, and lack of exposure to the sun may play a role in all types of depression, not just in the most serious seasonal-affective disorders, which tend to strike during winter months.

The sun/cancer link stems from research that found that women who live in the Northeast are 40 to 60% more likely to die from breast cancer than those who live in "sunnier" West Coast or southern areas. A new study by epidemiologist Ester John, PhD, at the Northern California Cancer Center, suggests that the incidence of cancer has as much to do with geography as with behavior. She found that women who lived in the South, or said that they were frequently outdoors, were 30 to 40% less likely to develop breast cancer than women who didn't fit that profile. Other research indicates that sunlight may help prevent prostate and colon cancers as well.

Experts attribute the lower risk to high levels of vitamin D, which the body produces when UVB rays penetrate the skin. Most of us don't get enough of this nutrient through diet alone. "If you live in the north, or are indoors a lot, you're at a greater risk for being vitamin D-deficient," says Susan Thys-Jacobs, MD, director of the Osteoporosis Center at St. Luke's Roosevelt Hospital in New York.

Recent evidence reveals that sunlight also stimulates the thyroid gland to increase hormone production, which increases metabolism, which means you'll burn up more energy or calories. In the excellent book *Sunlight,* author Zane Kime, MD, states, "There is conclusive evidence that exposure to sunlight produces a metabolic effect in the body very similar to that produced by physical training, and is definitely followed by a measurable improvement in physical fitness." He also explains in this book how a plant-based diet (vegan—no meat, dairy, or eggs) will greatly *decrease* the risk of skin cancer.

Just because a little bit of direct sunlight is great for your body doesn't mean that a lot is better. To allow sunburn is foolish. Immune-reacting systems are overstimulated by the action of too much sunlight, increasing body acidity. Dermatologists also prescribe caution regarding tanning beds. Nothing can match the benefits of natural sunlight. I have practiced safe sunning for over four decades—taught to me by my grandmother. Of course, baking in the sun is still not advisable, and morning and afternoon are better times to bask in the sun, especially during the summer. If you're in the sun longer than 20 or 30 minutes, apply a sunscreen with an SPF of at least 15 or above. But for those 10 to 20 minute sessions a few times a week, expose as much of your body to the sun as possible. If you can sunbathe "au natural," do it, as you'll reap more benefits of increased vitamin D and sex hormones when more skin is exposed. I usually do my aerobic workout outdoors in the form of morning hiking (clothed, of course!), allowing the sun to shine on my arms and face, and, when it's warm enough, on my legs. In this way, I get a great workout in a beautiful environment and reap the benefits of the healthy, early morning sunshine.

And speaking of exercise, this is the next tip for quelling stress and living with balance and vitality.

5. Exercise for life.

A majority of the year, I live in Los Angeles, the fitness capital of the world. People are so body conscious here, the first thing you might be asked when you meet someone is, "Have you got a good trainer and gym?" I wouldn't be surprised to start seeing ads in the personal columns that read: "Fit, trim, female weightlifter who bench-presses 150 pounds and has a cholesterol level of 150 looking for a tan, strong, toned man who has completed at least a dozen triathlons and has a triglyceride level of 75."

Of course, there are many reasons to stay in good shape beyond the fact that it's fashionable. Fitness is the key to enjoying life—it can unlock the energy, stamina, and positive outlook that make each day a pleasure. Along with good eating habits, adequate rest, enough sleep, and a positive attitude about yourself and life, exercise is an important facet of a total program for well-being. It is one of the commonsense ways to take responsibility for your own health and life.

Develop a well-rounded fitness program that includes strength training, aerobics, and stretching. Make your program a top priority in your life, a nonnegotiable activity, and stay committed to it. There is nothing that will do more good for you in terms of being vibrantly healthy, energetic, and youthful than a regular fitness program.

Never underestimate the benefits of regular aerobic exercise for cardio health. Just 30 minutes at least four times a week will help maintain a healthy weight and body-fat ratio while decreasing blood pressure, blood sugar, anxiety, depression, and insomnia. You need aerobic, or cardio, exercise to burn the fat out of your muscles. Then add strength training, or weight lifting, to build muscle which, in turn, increases metabolism. That's right, and it's that simple. Muscle burns fat. Proper exercise increases muscle, tones it, alters its chemistry, and increases its metabolic rate. More muscle means a faster metabolism because muscle uses more energy to exist than fat. Because muscle is a highly metabolic tissue, pound for pound it burns five times as many calories as most other body tissues. When you have more muscle mass, you burn more calories than someone who doesn't, even when you're both sitting still or sleeping. That's why people who build muscle have an easier time maintaining

> Develop a well-rounded fitness program that includes strength training, aerobics, and stretching.

a healthy weight. They're simply more efficient calorie burners. The addition of 10 pounds of muscle to your body will burn approximately 500 extra calories per day. You would have to jog 6 miles a day, 7 days a week to burn the same number of calories. Ten extra pounds of muscle can burn a pound of fat in one week—that's 52 pounds of fat a year!

To increase muscle, you must engage in strength training, such as weight lifting or other resistance training. All it takes to add 10 pounds of muscle is a regular strength training program involving 30 to 40 minutes, two to three times a week for about five to six months. Put simply, at least twice a week or more, strength train your chest, shoulders, arms, back, and legs for at least 30 minutes each session. Then add flexibility work (gentle stretching, yoga, or Pilates) to your cardio and weight-training routine, and you've completed the triangle of fitness. This triangle (cardio, weight training, and flexibility work) will reduce bone loss, maintain strength and muscle mass, and keep energy levels revved. Remember these three points: move, strengthen, and lengthen.

Regular physical exercise is also an effective means of reducing stress and tension. A single dose of exercise works better than tranquilizers as a muscle relaxant among people with symptoms of anxiety and tension, without the undesirable side effects. In a classic study of tense and anxious people, Herbert de Vries, PhD, former director of the Exercise Physiology Laboratory at the University of Southern California, administered a 400-mg dose of meprobamate, the main ingredient in many tranquilizers, to a group of patients. On another day, he had these same patients take a walk vigorous enough to raise their heart rates to more than 100 beats per minute. Using an EMG (electromyogram) machine to measure the patients' tension levels as shown by the amount of electrical activity in their muscles, de Vries found that after exercise the electrical activity was 20 percent less tense. By contrast, the same patients showed little difference after the dose of meprobamate.

Exercise physiologists and medical researchers are now discovering that our sense of happiness and well-being is greatly influenced by the presence of certain chemicals and hormones in the bloodstream.

Vigorous exercise stimulates the production of two chemicals that are known to lift the spirit—norepinephrine and enkephalin.

A British medical team headed by Dr. Malcolm Carruthers spent four years studying the effect of norepinephrine on two hundred people. Their conclusion: "We believe that most people could ban the blues with a simple, vigorous ten-minute exercise session three times a week. Ten minutes of exercise will double the body's level of this essential neurotransmitter, and the effect is long-lasting. Norepinephrine would seem from our research to be the chemical key to happiness."

Inactivity also leads to fatigue. According to the late Dr. Lawrence Lamb, former consultant to the President's Council on Physical Fitness and Sports, part of the reason for this has to do with the way we store adrenaline. Lamb reports, "Activity uses up adrenaline. If it isn't used, adrenaline saps energy and decreases the efficiency of the heart." The downward spiral of energy you feel at the end of the workday only will be worsened if you come home and collapse in an easy chair. "Exercise will get the metabolic machinery out of inertia," says Lamb, "and you'll be refreshed and ready to go."

If you would like more detailed information on exercise, when and how to do it, the best exercises for faster weight loss, and how to stay motivated, please refer to my book *Invest in Yourself with Exercise*, and also my Webinar of the same name, both featured on my website SusanSmithJones.com.

Another practice that will increase metabolism, boost your energy level, help alleviate mood swings, and reduce stress on your body is to graze throughout the day.

6. Eat more often and lose more weight.

Three meals a day, along with two or three low-calorie, nutrient-dense snacks between meals, will control hunger, stoke metabolism, and accelerate fat loss. This is referred to as grazing. It also reduces stress in the body because fewer meals (1 or 2) with the same number of calories as 5 to 6 smaller daily meals puts extra stress on the digestive system and all of the body's cells. The results of four national surveys show that most people try to lose weight by eating 1,000 to 1,500 calories a day. However, cutting calories to under 1,200 (if you're a woman) or 1,400 (if you're a man) doesn't provide a satisfying amount of food and slows down metabolism.

The typical dieter will often skip meals, especially breakfast. This temporary fasting state sends a signal to the body that food is scarce. As a result, the stress hormones increase and the body begins "lightening the load" and shedding its muscle tissue. Decreasing muscle tissue decreases the body's need for food. By the next feeding, the pancreas is sensitized and will sharply increase blood insulin levels, which is the body's signal to make fat. And if you're insulin resistant, as many sedentary people are, you make extra amounts of this hormone (insulin) and make/deposit fat very easily, especially if you eat refined carbohydrates. Have you ever wondered how sumo wrestlers get so big? They fast and then gorge themselves with food. As you can see, this approach is absolutely counterproductive if your goal is to lose fat and reduce stress in your body.

> If you want to increase your metabolism, it's best to eat several small, healthful meals each day.

If you want to increase your metabolism, it's best to eat several small, healthful meals each day, suggests Dean Ornish, MD, in his book, *Eat More, Weigh Less*. This kind of grazing approach to meals keeps your metabolism stoked. It also keeps you from feeling deprived—one of the chief complaints of everyone who has ever been on a diet.

We now know that eating smaller meals more often is good for muscle-building and weight loss. But did you know that it may even be an effective way to reduce high cholesterol? When researchers from the University of Cambridge, England, assessed data on more than 14,600 men and women ages 45 to 75, they found that those who ate 5 to 6 times daily had the lowest LDL ("bad") cholesterol levels. Those who dined only once or twice daily had the highest, on average.

As well, I like to take out 10 to 12 hours a day (on 2 to 3 days) of no eating at all except fresh vegetable juice and water (it's referred to as intermittent fasting), and for me, this is usually during the eight hours at night during which I am sleeping along with the hours before bed-time that I am not eating and the early morning hours before breakfast when I am engaging in my sacred time of prayer and meditation.

For one of your snacks during the day, have some fresh vegetable juice.

7. Heal with fresh vegetable juices.

Nothing is more healing and nutritious than fresh vegetable juices. Juices are concentrated nutritional elixirs that heal and rejuvenate the body and help bring balance to all the body's cells. Juicing is also one of the easiest, most efficient, and delicious ways to ensure you're meeting your daily produce quota.

Juicing is different from blending. When you juice, you separate the juice of the fruit or vegetable from the fiber. You might be thinking, "Why would I do that? Fiber is essential for good health." I agree and recommend both a high-fiber diet *and* fresh vegetable juices. The fiber found in raw vegetables, fresh fruits, and other plant-based foods (ani-mal products don't have any fiber) plays a vital role in the health of the colon, the promotion of regular bowel movements, and the transport of toxins out of the body. To maximize the benefits of raw foods and a whole-foods diet in general, we need a good balance of whole raw foods, as well as freshly extracted raw vegetable juice. To understand more clearly, here's a nutshell view of digestion.

The process of digestion begins in the mouth. Everything you eat is masticated (chewed), mixed with your salivary enzymes, and moved on to your stomach and intestines. Ultimately, the food is liquefied so that the nutrients can pass from the small intestines into the bloodstream and lymph fluid for distribution. The remaining fiber is passed into the colon for elimination after excess water and remaining minerals are absorbed. In other words, fresh juice provides pure nutrients that require little digestive effort for optimal utilization. The juicer does the digestive work in separating out the fiber, and we receive a treasure chest of nutrients in a form that's readily assimilated.

Today's commercial farming practices, topsoil erosion, and failure to let the land rest periodically mean lower nutrient density of our vegetables and fruits. Even eating the best raw fruits and vegetables may not be enough to insure an optimal level of health. In general, our bodies are malnourished, overfed, and dealing with a heavy load of internal toxicity. Our bodies are designed by God to be self-healing, self-renewing, and self-rejuvenating if we just give them the right ingredients, including emphasis on nutrients from raw, living foods. Juicing is a simple and efficacious way to maximize our nutrient intake without putting a heavy digestive burden on the body. It also helps the body eliminate toxins.

Decades ago, in one of my many visits with Bernard Jensen, PhD, he told me that by adding fresh juices to a balanced food regimen, you will help accelerate and enhance the process of restoring nutrients to chemically starved tissues. It is on these tissues that disease and illness thrive. In terms of prevention, therefore, the importance of juices cannot be overstated, he stated. In *Live Food Juices,* H. E. Kirschner, MD, says that if modern research is correct, the power to break down the cellular structure of raw vegetables and assimilate the precious elements they contain, even in the healthiest individual, is only fractional—not more than 35%, and in the less healthy, down to 1%. In the form of juices, he adds, these same individuals assimilate up to 92% of these elements.

Put simply, fresh juice is more than an excellent source of vitamins, minerals, enzymes, purified water, proteins, carbohydrates, and chlorophyll. Freshly made, because it's in liquid form, if drank on an empty stomach, supplies nutrition that is not wasted to fuel its own digestion as it is with whole fruits, vegetables, and grasses. As a result, your body's digestive system can quickly and easily make maximum use of all the nutrition that fresh juice offers.

> . . . your body's digestive system can quickly and easily make maximum use of all the nutrition that fresh juice offers.

Because of the higher sugar content of fresh fruit, I generally advocate eating whole fruit and juicing vegetables (in addition to eating lots of whole vegetables). I've been an avid juicer for about 50 years (learning about it from my grandmother when I was a child) and teach juicing in my healthy food preparation classes and in workshops around the world. In addition to making fresh vegetable juice often, I do an exclusive day of juice fasting once every week or two, and two to three consecutive days a month, consuming nothing but fresh vegetable juices, water, and my favorite teas. It's easy, fun, and provides the stamina I need to engage in my daily activities without necessitating much alteration of lifestyle. You just need a good juicer to take advantage of this superb health-promoting practice.

It takes about pound of carrots to make about a 10-ounce drink of carrot juice. But could you enjoy consuming that many carrots? Probably not. Yet all the enzymes, water-soluble vitamins, minerals, phytonutrients, and trace elements in those carrots are extracted (assuming it is a high-quality, slow-speed masticating juicer) and condensed into the glass of juice. The same thing applies to vegetables. You might have a hard time eating 4 to 7 servings of vegetables each day, but it's easy to consume the nutritional value of a variety of vegetables by juicing them.

In light of all the research on the benefits of fresh vegetable juices, it's difficult to understand why anyone would not favor the addition of fresh vegetable juices to their diet unless there is a misunderstanding about how efficiently the body handles the natural sugars in vegetable juices. Michael Donaldson, PhD, my friend and scientific director at Hallelujah Diet, conducted a study to determine the effect of carrot juice on blood glucose levels. He found, contrary to popular thinking, that the body actually handles the raw carrot juice very efficiently, with much less impact on the blood glucose than eating whole-grain bread. For people with blood sugar issues, adding a teaspoon of fresh flaxseed oil to the juice can further lower the glucose response to carrot juice.

Another option is to make the juice a combination of 40% carrot and 60% green leafy lettuce or other dark green vegetables. Here are just a few of the vegetables I juice: spinach, celery, beets, romaine lettuce, beets, Swiss chard, kale, collards, cauliflower, green onions, mustard greens, broccoli and broccoli sprouts, bell peppers, cabbage, and carrots. I also enjoy adding parsley, lemon, apple, garlic, and ginger. You'll find a variety of juicing recipes in my books and audio programs, which are available at SusanSmithJones.com.

Keep in mind that the more colorful, natural foods you eat, the healthier and more youthful you'll become.

8. Rejuvenate with colorful whole foods.

Of course, becoming healthy and balanced is more than merely choosing to eat wholesome, nutritious foods, but it's a good place to start. My approach to healthful eating is a diet of whole foods, as close as possible to the way Mother Nature has created them. It is this type of diet that restores harmony to the body, mind, and spirit and replenishes our body's life force. As my grandmother Fritzie taught me, food is a love note from God. What a glorious thought! In order to bring a sacred balance into our lives, we must choose foods that not only nourish all the cells of our body, but also feed our souls.

Our body is composed of over 70 trillion cells. Much of the fuel for our cells comes directly from the things we eat, which contain nutrients in the form of vitamins, minerals, water, carbohydrates, fats, proteins, and enzymes. Each nutrient differs in form and function, but all are vital. Nutrients are involved in every body process, from combating infection to repairing tissue to thinking. To eat is one of the most basic and powerful of human drives. Although eating has been woven into many cultural and religious practices, essentially we eat to survive.

> Even if you are not sick, you may not necessarily be healthy. It simply may be that you are not yet exhibiting any overt symptoms of illness.

The problem is that most of us simply do not get what we need from our modern diet. Even if you are not sick, you may not necessarily be healthy. It simply may be that you are not yet exhibiting any overt symptoms of illness. Unlike a car engine that immediately malfunctions if you put water into the gasoline tank, the human body has tremendous resilience and often camouflages the repercussions of unhealthy fuel choices.

It doesn't help that we are surrounded by bad influences when it comes to what we eat. We have come to believe that any combination of heated, treated, processed, chemicalized "foods" will meet our nutritional needs so long as we take plenty of vitamin pills, heartburn medicine, headache pills, laxatives, and other remedies. "Whether you're drawn to chocolate, cookies, potato chips, cheese, or burgers and fries," writes health researcher Neal Barnard, MD, in his book *Breaking the Food Seduction: The Hidden Reasons Behind Craving—and 7 Steps to End Them Naturally*, "we all have foods we can't seem to resist—foods that sabotage our best efforts. Banishing these cravings is *not* a question of willpower or psychology—it's a matter of biochemistry." Based on his research and that of other leading investigators at major universities, Dr. Barnard reveals the diet and lifestyle changes that can break these stubborn craving cycles—many of which are highlighted in this tip and many other of the 10 tips presented here.

Adding foods is easier than taking them away, and the simple addition to our diet of fresh fruits and vegetables will help protect the genes from being damaged. In fact, the heart of any quintessential diet is plenty of colorful, fresh produce. Driven by mounting scientific evidence, all the national health organizations, such as Dr. Barnard's PCRM (The Physician's Committee for Responsible Medicine), National Institutes of Health (NIH), and Hallelujah Diet have revised their dietary advice by putting a rainbow of fruits and vegetables front and center, where they belong. Fruits and vegetables are low in calories and high in nutrients, ideal foods for healing, vitality, weight loss, and alkalizing the body. Nature has color-coded them. A simple way to assure you're getting a healthy variety of nutrients is to enjoy an attractive panoply of colorful, natural foods.

> ... the simple addition to our diet of fresh fruits and vegetables will help protect the genes from being damaged.

My dear friend, Olin Idol, vice president of health at Hallelujah Diet, and I know that food is medicine. We've had many discussions about this over the decades. It was my grandmother who first taught me about the healing power of food when I was a teenager. Indeed, food is the most simple and effective form of drugs or prescriptions there is. When consuming the right nutrients, the natural, plant-based foods of the earth, the natural healing capabilities in our bodies kick into gear. Foods high in natural compounds found in a variety of fruits and vegetables can even have the power to fight cancer and disease.

Most people eat far too few foods with any color in them. Studies show that the average total intake of fruits and vegetables is about three servings daily (I recommend 7 to 12 servings daily). If those three servings are iceberg lettuce, french fries, and a little ketchup for color, you are in big trouble. Eating is pleasurable, and we have voted with our dollars for a beige diet of french fries, burgers, and cheese. The only problem with the diet we love is that it doesn't fit our genes, which evolved over eons in a plant-based, hunter-gatherer diet with half the fat, no dairy products, no processed foods, no refined sugars, no alcohol, and no tobacco.

Here is some food for thought—valuable information to enhance your brain function and improve memory. In 2004, the results from the Harvard Nurses Study extolled the virtues of eating green vegetables. Of the 13,000 women who participated, those who consumed at least 2½ cups of romaine lettuce and spinach per week (leafy greens) and 2½ cups of Brussels sprouts, cauliflower, and broccoli (cruciferous vegetables) were 1 to 2 years younger in brain function than those participants who eschewed these stellar foods. Your grandmother was right. If you want to be smarter, you need to eat your vegetables—especially lots of leafy greens.

The food choices you make today will determine the health you experience tomorrow. Think of food as something to nourish your body temple, to bring blessings to your life as you revel in the bounty that God provides. Just perusing the produce section of your grocery store can become a treasure hunt for you and your family. Encourage your children to go grocery shopping with you (being sure to stay only in the produce section) and then invite them to choose a different fruit or vegetable for the family to try. My best-selling nutrition book for children (coauthored with Dianne Warren), *Vegetable Soup/The Fruit Bowl*, teaches the connection between the foods they eat and how they look, think, feel, and perform. (You can order this book from my website: SusanSmithJones.com.)

Because fresh fruits and vegetables are the foods highest in water content, and because they are the foods easiest to digest, they take stress off your digestive system and are what I refer to as "body-friendly" foods, especially if you eat them in their raw, natural, organic state. Jettison processed and refined foods—anything made with white sugar or white flour—in favor of colorful, nutrient-dense, plant-based foods. According to Joel Fuhrman, MD, in his book, *Eat to Live,* "Americans have been among the first people worldwide to have the luxury of bombarding themselves with nutrient-deficient, high-calorie food, often called *empty-calorie* or *junk food.* [Empty-calorie means food that is deficient in nutrients and fiber.] More Americans than ever before are eating these rich, high-calorie foods while remaining inactive—a dangerous combination." I concur. And it's precisely for this reason that the number-one health problem in America and the United Kingdom is obesity.

In addition to selecting the most nutrient-dense foods to eat, I also encourage you to supplement your diet with fresh vegetable juices and natural food supplements (refer to my website for suggestions) to fill in any nutritional gaps. From Hallelujah Diet, I take their nutritious and delicious, raw BarleyMax powders every day (and they come in Original, Mint, and Berry—visit MyHDiet.com). Choosing to live a healthful lifestyle is a personal decision and something you must earn; you can't buy good health. Your health and happiness are inescapably linked. "Choose what is best; habit will soon render it agreeable and easy," opined Pythagoras more than 2,500 years ago. By eschewing disease-causing processed foods and switching over to a natural, whole foods diet—with an emphasis on colorful living (raw) foods, you will be providing nourishment for your body, mind, and spirit. What a gift to give your body and your loved ones—long life and enduring health. Without vibrant health, life loses its luster. As mentioned in Chapter 9, and bears repeating again, Ralph Waldo Emerson would probably agree. He gave us this true advice: "Health is our greatest wealth."

9. Fight cancer with a proven phytonutrient.

One reason for introducing more diversity of plant foods into our diets is that different foods provide different phytochemicals ("phyto" comes from the Greek work meaning *plant*). These plant chemicals have been proven to ward off disease and heal the body. One of these phytonutrients is salvestrol, which was inadvertently discovered only two decades ago by scientists who were looking for a way to keep normal cells healthy while treating cancer cells with medical drugs. Specifically, Gerry Potter, Professor of Medical Chemistry at De Montfort University in the United Kingdom, and Dan Burke, Professor Emeritus at North Carolina State University, discovered salvestrol in plants and then found that this natural substance could do exactly what they were hoping the drugs would do to cancer cells without the risks or potential reactions.

The published paper "Nutrition and Cancer: Salvestrol Case Studies" by Potter and Burke along with Brian Schaefer, DPhil, and Hoon Tan, PhD, explained what sets salvestrol apart from other phytonutrients: its direct relationship with cancer cells. Unlike other compounds, salvestrol has a connection with the enzyme found within cancer cells known for its tumor properties (CYP1B1). As reported in *Natural News* blog, when salvestrol is consumed from dietary plants, it helps the body to fight and kill cancerous cells by becoming metabolized by CYP1B1 while keeping healthy cells intact.

> **In addition to its cancer-fighting properties, salvestrol is also an antioxidant and an antimicrobial.**

The case studies discussed in the aforementioned paper used salvestrol supplementation along with changes in diet for melanoma, bladder cancer, prostate cancer, lung cancer, and breast cancer. The authors concluded that salvestrol and its metabolism by CYP1B1 create a "food-based rescue mechanism." Reporting that nutrition can greatly impact the outcomes for cancer patients, the authors advise the use of salvestrol alongside other strategies. In addition to its cancer-fighting properties, salvestrol is also an antioxidant and an antimicrobial. Like many phytonutrients, salvestrol likely works best in synergy with other nutrients found in abundance in a whole-foods, plant-based diet.

Today, it is harder for the body to get the necessary amount of salvestrol from plant foods needed to fight cancer. As the study authors explained, the evolution of processed foods has resulted in very low levels of natural phytonutrients, including salvestrol. In fact, they pointed to this as the potential cause of rising cancer rates. "Furthermore, modern agricultural methods have significantly depleted the salvestrol levels in our foods making it more and more difficult for us to benefit from this natural anticancer mechanism through diet alone," wrote the authors. This would explain why organic produce has been shown to contain 30% *more* salvestrol than nonorganic fruits and vegetables, according to the Underground Health Reporter. The agricultural and horticultural practices of today continue to strip the important phytonutrients from fruits, vegetables, and other natural foods. As such, choosing natural, whole, and unprocessed foods is the best way to gain optimal benefits.

Fruit sources high in salvestrol are grapes, strawberries, oranges, blueberries, black currants, tangerines, apples, and cranberries. Vegetables include cauliflower, broccoli, bell peppers, cabbage, Brussels sprouts, olives, and avocados. You can even get salvestrol through a number of herbs including sage, rosemary, mint, parsley, basil, and thyme, to name a few. For those who are battling cancer, supplementing with salvestrol may be another option. As the *Natural News* blog explained, doing so can help to reinstate that naturally occurring barrier—knocked down by modern toxins—against cancer.

The true power of salvestrol goes back to the original **Genesis 1:29** diet. As taught by the Hallelujah Diet organization, when we consume the plants of the earth as God intended, we are nourishing our bodies with the richest form of medicine, the most natural and nutritional substances there are. All the phytonutrients consumed from primarily raw, plant-based foods join forces to fight back together in synergy against foreign invaders like sickness, infection, and cancer. Unfortunately, over the years, the standard American diet (aka SAD) has gotten in the way and reduced these naturally occurring, powerful compounds from reaching the bodies of so many Americans.

While there is no singular answer to warding off disease, saying no to overly processed and packaged foods is an excellent place to start. From there, following a whole-foods diet with emphasis on plant-based foods, exercising regularly, drinking lots of water, and taking care of oneself as described in this book is following the path to optimal health. So while salvestrol can help fight cancer, it is important to keep in mind all the things attributed to a healthy lifestyle.

10. Look younger by the day with raw foods.

Scientists and doctors are now emphasizing the importance of fresh, raw foods in our diet due to the loss of essential vitamins, enzymes, friendly bacteria, and other important microorganisms caused by unnecessary cooking. Modern scientific medicine is finally catching up with traditional wisdom and helping us prevent the diseases caused by SAD, which you now know appropriately stands for the standard American diet.

The core philosophy of the raw food movement lies in the idea that enzymes, the catalysts needed to aid digestion and nutrient absorption, are destroyed at temperatures around 118°F. Enzymes remain intact within living foods below temperatures of 118°F (ideally 108°F). Higher temperatures destroy the enzymes, and our bodies have to work harder to digest the foods we consume. Enzyme-rich foods help provide our bodies with a more viable and efficient energy source. Raw foods rapidly digest in our stomach and begin to provide energy and nutrition at a quick rate. Consuming cooked food, either alone or before raw food, can cause a condition called leukocytosis, an increase in white blood cells. Your body may respond to cooked food as if it were a foreign bacteria or a diseased cell, which causes your immune system to waste energy on defending you. By eating only raw food or eating raw food before eating cooked food, you can prevent leukocytosis.

While the body also produces enzymes, some researchers believe that only a finite amount of them are available over the course of a lifetime. Raw theorists state that as the enzyme supply dwindles, the body ages more quickly, has less ability to fight disease, and essentially runs out of energy. Because raw food is in its original, natural form, it is more wholesome, assimilative, and digestible. Food eaten raw puts very little stress on the body's systems. Gabriel Cousens, MD, a raw foodist, recommends eating more raw foods for many reasons, the least of which is for their alkalinity, their high enzyme levels, and their ability to improve circulation. He says, "Live cell analysis experimentation has shown that within ten minutes after ingesting enzymes, red blood cells become un-clumped. Something is happening in the blood after the enzymes are ingested that suggests the enzymes are effective in the blood." In other words, the live enzymes in raw foods have a healing effect on the body.

> Your body may respond to cooked food as if it were a foreign bacteria or a diseased cell . . .

All food, like all matter, is vibrational energy. When we consume it, the vibration of the food is transferred to us as vital life force. Therefore, the fresher and more alive the food is, the more life force we receive. Most of us can't see this life force with our naked eye, but it can be measured by Kirlian photography. This remarkable form of electrophotography captures the energy field around living things, and double-blind studies have proven that awareness of this life force strengthens and magnifies the subtle energy even more. When volunteers in scientific experiments directed their healing energy into water, and the water was then given to plants, the plants responded by growing faster, larger, and more resistant to disease! We can do the same thing with our foods by focusing love energy into them as we prepare our meals. I have always loved preparing foods, and I consciously endeavor to bring my connection with nature and God into the kitchen with me.

I find that raw food provides a far greater range of taste than cooked food. The most popular misconception is that raw food is all one texture: crunch. People don't understand that there is a whole range of textures, such as creamy and chewy. This food can be warm or cold or just cool: the right spices add heat and excitement.

As a proponent of a raw foods diet, I've emphasized eating raw foods for years and teach courses in "Living Food Cuisine." Participants new to this way of eating and living—it's more a lifestyle, not just a "diet"—are always astounded at how great they feel after a few days on raw foods. When people reduce the amount of cooked food in favor of more colorful raw foods, like fresh fruits and vegetables, they see tremendous positive changes in their health. I have seen major turnarounds with clients and friends in cancer, heart disease, diabetes, hypoglycemia, thyroid disorders, hormone imbalance, weight problems, and many other health struggles just by adding in more raw foods to the diet. After seeing all these benefits, I am completely convinced there is *something very powerful and profound* to raw foods.

The changes I've seen after eating more raw foods go beyond physical to the mental, emotional, and spiritual. I experience more inner peace, joy, harmony, and clarity. My eyes become clearer and more violet-blue, extra weight falls away, my skin becomes softer, wrinkles abate, and people tell me that I look younger. I have more energy throughout the day, can eat all day long without gaining weight, and feel a deeper connection with my own Divinity and connectedness with all life and God. That's why I often refer to it as spiritual nutrition. All you have to do is try this for 30 days, and you'll see the difference. It's hard to put into words the feeling of balance, well-being, and personal power you experience when eating all or a mostly raw-food diet. The claims of rejuvenating effects are almost universal in raw food communities.

Elisabetta Politi, head of nutrition at Duke University Diet & Fitness Center, says that any way of eating that promotes minimal food processing needs to be looked at seriously. "I think people would benefit from having more raw foods in a well-balanced diet," she says, while cautioning that an entirely raw diet would be very difficult to sustain for most of the population.

I'm the first to admit that living 100% raw is not an easy thing to do when you need to integrate into "normal" society. And I also don't suggest that you switch your diet from all or mostly cooked to all raw foods overnight. In my books and workshops, I recommend beginning with adding 50% raw food to each meal. For example, you might add a juice or a smoothie with breakfast or add in a generous portion of fresh fruit to your cereal. For lunch, include a garden salad with your sandwich (and lots of vegetables on the sandwich) and a different salad at dinner with other cooked food. For your snacks, try some fresh fruit, vegetable juice, cut-up raw vegetables, trail mix, or some raw fruit and seed pudding (made with chia seeds—refer to the recipe for "Vanilla Chia Seed Pudding" at the end of Chapter 17) or raw vegetable soup.

As mentioned, when eating cooked food, always start with a few bites of raw food first. Or upgrade the 50% raw regimen to include two days a week with raw meals as many of my clients do. Maybe on a Monday you eat only raw foods all day until dinner when you have 50% raw (24 hours on raw). Then on Thursday incorporate 36 hours on raw—all day Thursday through Friday morning. Weekdays seem to be easier than weekends for most of my clients.

If you have no desire to eat a totally raw-food diet, I encourage you to aspire to at least 60%, or better yet, 85% raw foods. From my experience, having worked with thousands of people, it seems that this higher amount of raw food versus cooked food will make a profound difference in how you feel and look. I am not a "raw-food purist." I still enjoy cooking and going out to eat, but most of the time, I consume healthful raw foods. Remember, raw doesn't necessarily mean cold. Foods may be warmed to well above body temperature and still maintain their life force. A good rule of thumb is: If you stick your finger in it, it should feel warm—not hot.

At the end of tip #15, you will find a story about one of my clients, Daniella, who changed the diet of her family and it had a myriad of healthful benefits.

11. Upgrade your vitality with soothing heat therapy.

Throughout this book, I've mentioned briefly the importance of using an infrared sauna. Here's more detail since it's one of two most important healthy-living practices in my life (along with drinking homemade, fresh alkaline water from my Ionizer Plus device—both from the High Tech Health [HTH] Company in Boulder, CO.)

For thousands of years, cultures throughout the world have enjoyed the many therapeutic benefits of saunas. They've recognized that sauna sessions help to rid the body of toxins, aid weight loss, kill viruses, beautify skin, ease achy joints and muscles, relax the body, and more. However, not all saunas are alike. Many scientific studies show that we get the most benefit from an infrared sauna as compared to the traditional dry sauna or the steam room. Please refer to my website (SusanSmithJones.com) to learn about these different types.

> . . . a person can burn up to 300 calories during one sauna session, the equivalent of a two- to three-mile jog or an hour of moderate weight training.

Want to lose weight? Studies show that a person can burn up to 300 calories during one sauna session, the equivalent of a two- to three-mile jog or an hour of moderate weight training. The infrared sauna creates a "fever" reaction that kills potentially dangerous viruses and bacteria and increases the number of leukocytes in the blood, thereby strengthening the immune system—important for fighting colds, flu, cancer, and bolstering resistance to infections. In other words, it increases and accelerates the body's own healing activity and restorative capacity.

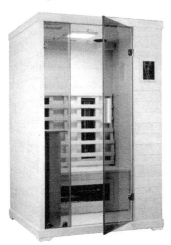

Every home should have a personal infrared sauna—and you want only the best, handcrafted one with environmentally safe wood, EMF-free heaters, and more. For over 20 years, I have used and highly recommend the Transcend Infrared Sauna by HTH (**800-794-5355** or **303-413-8500, ext. 2** or visit **HighTech-Health.com**), which comes in different sizes. Under "Favorite Products" on my website, you'll find many of my articles posted with detailed info on heat therapy and how infrared saunas heal us head-to-toe. Call and ask them any questions you may have and how to get a substantial discount on your purchase (use my name "SSJ" as a code). This Transcend is the best infrared sauna in the industry—and you deserve the best!

12. Practice the art of relaxation and deep breathing.

One of the world's leading experts on the brain is a former Harvard medical doctor, Herbert Benson, MD, author of *The Relaxation Response* and *Your Maximum Mind*, and briefly mentioned in Chapter 8. What Benson calls "the relaxation response" is the body's ability to enter into a state characterized by an overall reduction of the metabolic rate and a lowered heart rate. According to Benson, this state of relaxation also acts as a door to a renewed mind, a changed life, and a feeling of awareness. He describes the physiological changes that occur when you are relaxed as a harmonizing or increased communication between the two sides of the brain, resulting in feelings often described as well-being, unboundedness, infinite connection, and peak experience.

One way to cultivate calmness and peacefulness is to progressively relax your body, beginning with your toes and ending with your head. Breathe slowly and deeply, and totally relax each part of your body, saying to yourself as you go along, "My toes, feet, legs [and so on] are relaxed," until you have gone through your entire body. Then rest for a while in the quiet and silence. Listening to a relaxation or meditation recording also may be helpful. (You can find out more about my own relaxation audio programs by visiting my website.)

Here's another great tip you can easily do at work or at home to help relax your mind and body. Look at a picture of a beautiful landscape. Yes, it's that simple! Two studies measured the effect of certain photographic images on emotional and physiological responses. The first study was designed to find ways of fighting the boredom and homesickness that astronauts experience during extended stays in space. Researchers projected a variety of slides on the walls of a room built to simulate a space station and recorded the subjects' responses to various scenes. The second study focused on hospital patients who were about to undergo surgery. In both groups, pictures of spacious views and glistening water lowered heart rates and produced feelings of calmness.

An easy and inexpensive way to look at a beautiful landscape is to get a poster. I have a framed Sierra Club poster in my meditation corner of my bedroom that has a dazzling view of water, mountains, and colorful wildflowers. Every time I look at it, I feel more relaxed. This is the perfect solution if you work in an office without windows. Larger posters of resplendent nature scenes can transform a room and provide you with a mini-fantasy vacation whenever you need it.

I also highly recommend getting one of those "sound soothers" that offer a variety of nature sounds, everything from gentle rain, to ocean waves, and a flowing brook, to a waterfall, an aviary, and windchimes. I use mine daily.

With regard to deep breathing, can you breathe your way to vibrant health? In most cases, I think you can. How often do you pause to consider the intricacies of breathing? Breathing is perhaps the only physiological process that can be either voluntary or involuntary. One can breathe, making their breath do whatever they wish, or one can ignore it, and after a while the body simply begins to breathe on its own. Breathing becomes reflexive. The body can't operate without breathing, so if conscious control of the breath is abandoned, then some unconscious part of the mind begins function-

> Breathing is perhaps the only physiological process that can be either voluntary or involuntary.

ing, picks it up, and starts breathing for us. Something is triggered in the lower part of the brain. But in this case, breathing falls back under the control of primitive parts of the brain, the unconscious realms of the mind, where emotions, thoughts, and feelings (of which we may have little or no awareness) become involved. These wreak havoc with breath rhythms. In other words, the breath becomes haphazard and often irregular if we lose conscious control of it. It's important to bring breath back into your awareness so it's reintegrated into your conscious-ness. This is one of the reasons I recommend in Chapter 8 to slowly and deeply inhale and exhale as you undertake the sacred prayer-meditation affirmations I provided (or make up your own).

Are your breaths rapid and shallow? Take a minute now (60 sec-onds) to check and see how many breaths per minute you take (count both the inhalation and exhalation as one breath). If it is between 16 and 20, then you are most likely a thoracic breather. This means that your breaths are not getting to the lower part of your lungs but remain fairly high in the chest. Thoracic breathing is the least efficient and most common type.

Diaphragmatic or deep abdominal breathing, on the other hand, promotes a more relaxed state. Take a long, slow, deep breath right now. Visualize the air filling the lower part of the lungs. Since gravity pulls more blood into that area, the most efficient passage of oxygen into the blood occurs there, slowing the breath as the body gets more oxygen. It's important to note how closely tied are respiration and the heart. As the breath slows (to 6 to 8 breaths per minute) and deepens, the heart's job is made considerably easier. There is evidence to suggest that diaphragmatic breathing is beneficial because it increases the suction pressure created in the thoracic cavity and improves the venous return of blood, thereby reducing the load on the heart and enhancing circulatory function. Also, diaphragmatic breathing has the added bonus of relaxing the muscles of the ribs, chest, and stomach.

Diaphragmatic breathing is really quite simple. It's the habit of doing it that must be consciously cultivated before it can become automatic. A simple practice to achieve this is to lie on your back on your bed or a mat or rug, with one palm placed on the center of the chest and the other on the lower edge of the rib cage where the abdomen begins. As you inhale, the lower edge of the rib cage should expand and the abdomen should rise; as you exhale, the opposite should occur; there should be relatively little movement of the upper chest. By practicing diaphragmatic breathing, you will find in time that this exercise is becoming habitual and automatic.

So choose to cultivate the habit of deep breathing. To make deep breathing automatic in my life, I tried this experiment several years ago: I set my watch to beep every hour (except when I was sleeping, of course), and I took one to three minutes to do some deep breathing. As the days and weeks went on, I noticed that when the hourly beep came around, I was already practicing deep breathing; it was increasingly becoming a habit. Now, most of the time, diaphragmatic breathing is my natural way to breathe.

Simply put: Developing harmonious and rhythmic breathing along with diaphragmatic breathing will have health benefits and can improve your quality of life. But even the best diaphragmatic breathing cannot stop the cellular aging process. As you age, your cells become less able to use the oxygen in the air to generate cell energy. My advice is to optimize your breathing and enhance the air you breathe with Molecular Hydrogen Therapy (a molecular hydrogen inhaler device), which I mentioned earlier in the book. Breathing in this salubrious mixed gas air daily promotes cell vitality, better mental and physical performance, healthy and slower aging, and repair for the damage of excessive free radicals. For more information on molecular hydrogen inhalers, go to "Favorite Products" on my website SusanSmithJones.com to find many articles on the topic and where to purchase the tablets or breathing device.

I have always found that when I'm relaxed, calm, and balanced and have been breathing deeply on a regular basis, it's easier to live in the moment and laugh at myself and all the incongruities of daily life.

13. Be in the precious present and laugh often.

Living *in* the moment is different from living *for* the moment. Young children seem to be masters of getting totally involved in and focused on whatever they are doing right now. Granted, their attention span is not long, but they are able to focus on whatever is taking place in their lives at the moment. When they eat, they just eat; when they play, they just play; when they talk, they just talk. They throw themselves wholeheartedly into their activities.

Have you ever noticed that young children are willing to try anything at a moment's notice? Even though they might have experienced that same thing before, they will express wide-eyed excitement and wonderment. Children don't use a yardstick to measure activities or compare the present with the past. They know they've played the game before, or had someone read the same story just last night, yet the game or the story is still as fresh and as wonderful as it was the first time.

Think about your attitude when doing the dishes, vacuuming, or watering the plants. You probably find these activities boring. But a child can't wait to participate, and acts as though it's just about the most exciting thing he or she has ever done. What a wonderful quality that is! To be excited about life—about every part of life as though it's always fresh and new. Actually, it is. It's only old thoughts and distorted attitudes that get in the way of celebrating each moment.

One way to be mindful of the present moment is to focus on your breathing, as elucidated earlier. "Conscious breathing, which is a powerful meditation in its own right," writes Eckhart Tolle in the book *The Power of Now*, "will gradually put you in touch with the body. Follow the breath with your attention as it moves in and out of your body. Breathe into the body, and feel your abdomen expanding and contracting slightly with each inhalation and exhalation. If you find it easy to visualize, close your eyes and see yourself surrounded by God's light or immersed in the light-filled arms of Jesus or the luminescent wings of your guardian angels. Then breathe in that light." I do this exercise a few times each day to help me remember to be in the present moment.

> "When your attention is in the present moment, you enjoy life more intensely because you are fully alive."

This precious present moment is the only moment we'll ever have. It's our moment of power and all there is in life. In this moment, problems do not exist. It is here we find our joy and balance and are able to embrace our authentic self and our oneness with God, with Spirit. It is here we discover that we are already complete and perfect, according to Tolle. If we are able to be fully present and take each step in the "Now," we will be opening ourselves to the transforming experience of the power of the present. "When your attention is in the present moment, you enjoy life more intensely because you are fully alive," writes Don Miguel Ruiz in another one of my favorite books, *The Four Agreements*. I like that a lot. You enjoy life more intensely because you are fully alive! How alive and present are you to the Now in your life?

Have you ever driven to work or run errands and not remembered how you got there? Check in with yourself every hour or so. Are you slouching? How's your attitude? What are you thinking? Is your breathing shallow? Don't wait until your shoulders are up around your ears before you try to relax. Learn to be mindful about how you're feeling and what's happening around you. I usually describe mindfulness as developing the mind's capacity to attain a balanced, awake understanding of what's happening, knowing how you feel about it, and choosing your wisest response. In my estimation, your wisest response—no matter what's going on in your life at the moment—is to embrace a cheerful attitude.

With regard to laughter, along with my faith in God, meditation/prayer time, being in nature, and living in the present moment, laughter is another one of my favorite ways to mollify stress. It is okay to laugh, even when times are tough. Toxic worry almost always entails a loss of perspective; a sense of humor almost always restores it.

It was the late Norman Cousins, a noted journalist, author, and my friend who, during a life-threatening illness, was able to achieve two hours of pain-free living for every ten minutes he devoted to laughter. In his renowned book, *Anatomy of an Illness*, he told about how he watched old comedies by the Marx Brothers and the Three Stooges and *Candid Camera* by the hour. He learned that laughter—hearty belly laughter—produced certain chemicals in the brain that benefit body, mind, and emotions.

According to researchers, as mentioned in the first intermission in this book, laughter releases endorphins into the body that act as natural stress beaters. Laughter also aids most—and probably all—major systems of the body. A good laugh gives the heart muscles a good workout, improves circulation, fills the lungs with oxygen-rich air, clears the respiratory passages, stimulates alertness hormones that stimulate various tissues, and alters the brain by diminishing tension in the central nervous system. It also helps relieve pain and counteracts fear, anger, and depression—all of which are linked to physical illness and stress.

Just recently, the results of a scientific study on the power of laughter were trumpeted on all the major television news stations. The study results disclosed that it only takes *one minute of laughter to boost the immune system for 24 hours! And one minute of anger suppresses immunity for six hours!* The elixir of life—and the best way to soften your heart and diminish the wrinkles around your soul (and on your face!)—is hearty laughter. Laughter is a sterling stress buster and loving gift we can give ourselves and others in our lives. Laughter is calorie- and pain-free and costs nothing; the dividends are priceless.

Another superlative way to relieve pain and depression, improve circulation, reduce stress, and help balance your body and life is through massage.

14. Enjoy time in God's resplendent nature.

Being out in nature, where the air is filled with healthy negative ions, lifts the spirits, relaxes the body, and gives us a sense of well-being. The air all around us is electrically charged with positive and negative ions. Most of us live and work in environments dominated by technology—surrounded by computers, microwaves, air conditioners, heaters, TVs, and vehicular traffic. These and other "conveniences" of modern life emit excessive amounts of positive ions into the air we breathe, which can result in mental or physical exhaustion and affect overall wellness. But when you're in nature, especially surrounded by water—like the ocean or a stream or lake—or in a forest of green trees, negative ions abound. In fact, the revolving water generated by fountains creates negative ions that cause air particles to achieve electrical (ionic) balance.

One way to increase the negative ions in your environment is to surround yourself with fountains. I have them all over my home—in my gardens and in several rooms—running 24/7 except in the bedroom, where I prefer quiet when sleeping. Since ancient times, the sound created by moving or flowing water has been known to have great healing power. (Refer to Chapter 9 to see how flowing water can help you increase your abundance and prosperity.) It has been said that the movement of water releases negative ions (chi energy), which, in turn, makes you feel refreshed, bringing peace to your heart and mind.

One of my favorite activities is hiking in my local Santa Monica Mountains early in the morning. When hiking you can take in a variety of terrain, flora, and fauna, while soaking up a wide range of sensations, sights, sounds, and scents as you move and work out your entire body. Hiking strengthens your body and feeds your soul, and you feel invigorated throughout the day.

We can learn so much from Mother Nature. She shows us the rhythm of the seasons and the balance of existence; the importance of times of withdrawal in attaining peace and serenity; the necessity of acceptance—flowing with the conditions of life; the wise use of energy and play; the true freedom that comes from lack of self-consciousness; and the strength that comes from being totally in the present.

One thing I know for sure. I always feel more positive and filled with gratitude when I spend quality time out in nature, which is the forthcoming Tip #15.

With regard to earthing or grounding, to explain it in a nutshell, we are electro-chemical organisms. Most of the biological processes in our body are driven by differences in electrical potential across cellular membranes. When we are connected (or grounded) to the earth, we are connected to the earth's electrical field, and benefit from what is known as the *grounding effect*. The earth has a net negative charge, and when our bare feet come into contact with the earth's surface (aka grounding), electrons are able to flow freely from the earth into our bodies.

> When we are connected (or grounded) to the earth, we are connected to the earth's electrical field . . .

This effect of grounding/earthing neutralizes the buildup of positive charges in our bodies. If you've ever shuffled across a carpet and touched a doorknob, then you've seen firsthand how an electric charge can build up in our bodies, and be released when we contact a grounded source. A grounding mat functions similarly.

In the modern world, we spend most of our time in insulated rubber shoes. The rubber in shoes is not conductive, and cuts us off from the earth. Lack of contact with the earth coupled with life in a modern technological environment means that we are constantly bombarded with electromagnetic fields. Leading EMF researcher Dr. Martin Pall has said that electromagnetic fields directly impact us at the cellular level by activating voltage-gated calcium channels, particularly in cardiac and neural tissues. Unwanted activation of these channels can result in myriad negative health symptoms, including pain and inflammation.

Losing our shoes and grounding by walking barefoot on the earth's surface or via a grounding pad or earthing mat allows the free flow of health-enriching electrons into our bodies. These electrons neutralize positive charges built up over the course of time. Earthing products, particularly grounding mats, have become increasingly popular as the science of grounding evolves. More research is showing incredible benefits of grounding therapy all the time. In a perfect word, we could get all the benefits of earthing by spending our days barefoot outside. Unfortunately, we spend most of our time indoors (and in shoes!), and the modern urban environment is not really conducive to barefoot activity. A grounding mat is a safe, effective, and convenient alternative that can be used anywhere, any time.

As I am writing this section of the book at my desk, and whenever I am at my desk, I put my bare feet on a grounding mat. This kind of mat plugs into the ground port of any electrical outlet, connecting you instantly to the earth's electric field. Placing your bare feet (or any exposed skin) on a grounding pad can effectively disperse any accumulated electric charge. Studies have shown that connection with the earth's negative charge allows the free flow of electrons into the body. These electrons may act in an antioxidant capacity, neutralizing harmful free radicals. Other studies have shown potential benefits for hormone regulation, blood flow and cardiovascular disease, mood, sleep, pain, and chronic inflammation.

Enjoy the benefits of grounding therapy at home today with your own grounding mat! The best one is from the company Vital Reaction, a sister company to High Tech Health in Boulder, CO, where I purchased mine. I give them as gifts to people often and they are always amazed at how much better they feel once using this mat.

And when you are using this mood-uplifting mat and you are feeling so happy and positive, it's a great time to think about all the things for which you are grateful.

15. Cultivate an attitude of gratitude.

Choose to be positive and grateful every day. The link between mind and body has been contemplated since the time of Plato, but it's only recently that research has been done on the neurophysiology of the brain. *Every* thought transmits instructions to the body through some 70 trillion nerve cells, so when you think a negative thought, your immune system is immediately compromised. By the same token, when you think positive thoughts, your immune system is enhanced and your whole body benefits. Furthermore, an anxious or fearful mind instructs the body to be likewise—tense and nervous. A calm mind creates a calm body.

Keep your thoughts imbued with your highest vision of how you'd like to live and what you want to experience in life. In other words, visualize your goals and dreams. Dream big! Regardless of circum-

> "You are never given a wish without also being given the ability to make it come true."

stances, always be persistent and keep the faith because *you can create your heart's desires.* You are full of infinite possibilities; whatever you can imagine, you can accomplish. **Romans 8:28**: *All things work together for good to and for those who love God.* **2 Corinthians 4:7**: *You already have within you the excellent power of God; you just need to stir it up and release it.* **Luke 1:37**: *For with God, nothing will be impossible.* Similarly, in his books *Jonathan Livingston Seagull* and *Illusions,* author Richard Bach writes that you are never given a wish without also being given the ability to make it come true. And it was the mythologist Joseph Campbell who offered the following exquisite advice: *Follow your bliss.* When I pay attention to and honor the stirrings of my heart and soul, I look and feel younger. We age quickly when we live with regret instead of cultivating our highest visions and dreams.

So choose your thoughts wisely. A new report from the *Mayo Proceedings* suggests that individuals who profess pessimistic explanations for life events have poorer physical health and a higher mortality rate compared with either optimists or "middle-of-the-road" types, regardless of age or sex. In fact, every 10-point increase in the study's pessimism scores was associated with a 19% increase in the risk of death. Conversely, participants whose test scores indicated optimism had a survival rate significantly better than expected. The reason for this may be that pessimists may be more "passive" or have a "darker" outlook on life than other personality types, leaving them more prone to bad life events—such as illness, injury, and depression. The researchers concluded that pessimism itself is a "risk factor" for early death, and should be viewed in the same way as other risk factors, such as obesity, high blood pressure, or high cholesterol level.

When you find one thing, however small, for which to be thankful, and you hold that feeling for as little as *15 seconds*, research reveals that many subtle and beneficial physiologic changes take place in your body, including the following four:

1. Stress hormone levels of cortisol and norepinephrine decrease, creating a cascade of beneficial metabolic changes such as an enhanced immune system.

2. Coronary arteries relax, thus increasing the blood supply to your heart.

3. Heart rhythm becomes more harmonious, which positively affects your mood and all other bodily organs.

4. Breathing becomes deeper, thus increasing the oxygen level of your tissues.

If all of this happens when you focus for just 15 seconds on something that brings you pleasure, joy, or a feeling of gratitude, imagine what would happen to your health if you were able to cultivate grateful thoughts and feelings regularly, at least once per hour throughout each day of the year. The health benefits of gratitude (which is really the same thing as love) are an amazing example of how connected the bridge between the mind, body, and emotions really is and how simple it is to put this connection to work in your own life. But, as you well know, simple isn't necessarily easy. Like everything important in life, you must make a conscious choice and take action.

Gratitude (and appreciation) is a magnetic force that draws more good to each one of us. It's a dynamic spiritual energy that allows you to exert a powerful influence on your body, life, and world. Most importantly, it's a stellar stress buster. What you think about consistently, you bring about in your life. Keep a gratitude journal and each day write down at least three things for which you are grateful. Focusing on the positive things, even during the most difficult times, is the perfect remedy to reduce and alleviate stress. And if you don't feel positive and grateful, "fake it until you make it," as the saying goes. In other words, "acting as if" will help you through many challenging times and carry you on to better times. It was Shakespeare who championed this sage advice in his immortal words in *Hamlet:* "Assume a virtue, if you have it not."

One of the countless things I'm grateful for in my life is my friendships with others and being blessed with so many wonderful clients. I treasure the feeling of being surrounded by tenderhearted people. So here's a story of one of my clients and how making some lifestyle changes enriched the quality of her life and also with her husband and children.

Daniella's Story: Change Your Diet, Change Your Life

Daniella is a great example of how changing our diet and adding more living, whole foods can not only assist with weight loss but also improve every aspect of family life and self-esteem. Married, with three children ages five, eight and twelve, Daniella initially came to me for motivation and help in losing some fat, toning up her body, and increasing her energy. As a first step, I asked her to keep a seven-day food diary and record exactly what and when she ate. Like all my new clients, she was instructed not to eat differently simply because I would be looking at the list; she had to be honest and write down everything, because there's no other way to make a true evaluation.

When I received her food diary, it was quite apparent why she had gained almost 30 pounds in 18 months and always felt enervated. Her diet was about 60% fat, the carbohydrates she consumed were almost all refined, she usually skipped breakfast because she was too busy getting the kids ready for school, and she always ate late at night. Her diary came straight out of my "encyclopedia of deleterious habits"! She rarely included raw foods in her diet, or her family's, explaining that it took too long to chew the food and she didn't have time. Daniella also noted that her kids disliked raw foods, so only on rare occasions did she have a few fruits and vegetables in the house. (Her youngest child loved my colorful 2-in-1 nutrition book for children ages 1 to 8 titled *Vegetable Soup/The Fruit Bowl,* coauthored with Dianne Warren, and, as a result of reading it often, she started eating—and even enjoying—healthier foods. For more information on this book or to purchase, please visit SusanSmithJones.com.)

As I inquired more about her family life, routines, eating habits, and so on, I learned that all her children were on the heavy side. The oldest girl was starting to be ridiculed in school because of her size. Not surprisingly, Daniella told me that her husband also needed to lose about 50 pounds. His blood pressure, cholesterol, and triglycerides were much too high and his doctor had suggested that he go on a diet. I told Daniella that no diet was necessary. Her family needed a health makeover, and I assured her that she had come to the right person for guidance.

My initial evaluation of how they ate and lived led me to suggest something very out of the ordinary. Knowing that they had a very large house with a guest room next to the kitchen, I asked if I could stay with them from Thursday through Saturday night. I wanted to experience their lifestyle as a family, to see how they lived at home, when and what they ate, and how they spent their time when not eating, in order to coach them in a healthier way of living. Yes, I brought most of my own food, and I simply observed like a butterfly on the wall (I like butterflies better than flies) and took lots of notes. I had Daniella's permission, when they were out of the house, to look through their pantry and refrigerator and all their kitchen cupboards. Sure enough, I found hardly any fresh, whole foods.

At mealtime, everyone salted the food before tasting it, and their dining table was never without canned sodas or processed fruit juices, butter, sour cream, and mounds of cheese. All five of them ate their meals quickly, without much conversation and without putting the utensils down between bites. Much overeating may be unintentional, since many popular foods contain hidden sugar and oils put there to stimulate the taste buds, and this was definitely the case with Daniella's family.

With Daniella's consent, I made a clean sweep of her kitchen. The rest of her family went along, although they were far from enthusiastic. I removed all refined carbohydrates, including pasta, white rice, low-fiber cereals, pancake and cookie mixes, white breads and bagels, and gave them to a homeless shelter. I replaced these with high-fiber breads and whole grains. I also rid their kitchen of margarine, mayonnaise, and vegetable shortenings and oils. Next, I gave away all the whole milk and cheese products. Those high-fat, calorie-loaded cheese slices provide between 80 and 140 calories per one-ounce slice, depending on the fat content. I replaced the whole milk with raw nut and seed milks; it turned out that they all loved the vanilla-flavor almond beverage the best after about two weeks of adapting to the new taste.

I took the entire family to the nearest health food store, showed them all the healthy alternatives such as veggie burgers and whole-grain pastas and, to the amazement of all of them, let them experience the produce section of the store. They were enthralled by all the colors and varieties of fruits and vegetables, many of which they had never seen before. We started with some of the most familiar—organic apples, oranges, pears, grapes, bananas, and strawberries.

In place of sodas and other canned drinks, I taught them how to make their own juice. The kids loved juicing and actually wanted to take it over as their daily job. Of course, I encouraged them to start drinking more water. Daniella's husband confessed to me secretly that he couldn't remember having more than about six glasses of water weekly. When I told him that I drink half of my body weight in ounces of purified, alkaline water every day, he almost collapsed in shock!

Yes, it took about one month for the family to adjust their taste buds to the new flavors, textures, and colors of their foods. They basically switched from a white and beige diet to a banquet of rainbow colors. Almost half of their diet was now raw foods, with an abundance of fresh fruits and vegetables. When you fill up on these salubrious foods, you nourish your body and actually lose much of your desire for junk or other processed foods.

After three months, it was time to introduce them to the benefits of consuming more raw foods and also showed them several simple raw-food recipes they could enjoy often. They were eager to move in that direction. After several un-cooking lessons, Daniella found it wasn't so hard to cook healthier meals. The entire family loved my recipe for fiber-rich and delicious raw chia seed pudding (see page 251 for the recipe).

As a result of eating more fiber and more nutritious foods, the family all lost weight, had more energy and balanced moods and a greater sense of well-being that resulted in more positive attitudes all around. I encouraged them all to be more active instead of hanging out in front of televisions or computers most nights and weekends, and their higher activity resulted in sounder sleep for everyone. Daniella's oldest daughter lost weight and joined an after-school sports team, which ended the ridicule and helped her self-esteem soar.

It's truly remarkable how making a few basic changes in one's diet can profoundly affect every area of life. The change this family had the hardest time with initially, but which ultimately turned out to be the most fun, was the one day each week of raw food. Remember, when I first met them, about 95% of their diet was all cooked foods. So, I suggested they not pick a weekend day but rather a Tuesday, Wednesday, or Thursday. They selected Thursday and from morning through evening ate only living foods—lots of fruits and vegetables, salads, and a variety of other fun foods, including nut butters, sprouts, sauces, soups—even cookies and other desserts. The family came to appreciate Daniella's gift for experimenting and creating new raw-food meals. A few weeks into their new health regimen, they started having friends over for meals to sample their delicious "health nut food!"

As I mentioned earlier, even though you may not be eager to overhaul your entire food program, at least start by adding more raw enzyme-rich organic fruits and vegetables to your diet. I recommend the following program to my clients and friends. Make at least 60% of your diet raw each and every day (85% is even better). On Mondays, eat raw foods all day until dinner, and on Thursdays, raw foods all day *including* dinner. This simple program will assist you to bring more living foods into your diet by spacing them out over the week. You'll feel lighter and more energetic immediately, simply from eating more uncooked foods.

Daniella followed her heart, which was guiding her in the direction of a healthier and more rewarding life for her and her family. She listened to her inner voice, which is the final tip on how to enrich the quality of your life.

16. Listen to your inner voice.

Have you ever been thinking of someone you haven't heard from in a long time when suddenly that person called? Did you ever have the feeling that a friend was in trouble, and then contacted her and found out that she was, indeed? Or have you ever met someone and somehow known that this person was going to be your spouse? Some call it a sixth sense, a hunch, a gut feeling, going on instinct, or just knowing deep inside. Psychologists call it intuition—an obscure mental function that provides us with information so that we know without knowing how we know. I refer to it as God talking to us and giving us direction. It was Ralph Waldo Emerson who said: "Let us be silent that we may hear the whispers of God."

> . . . as we pay attention to our intuition and act on what we hear or feel, we reduce stress and create more balance in our lives.

How tuned-in are you to this voice within? When you get a message, do you usually write it off as nothing? I have found from countless experiences that as we pay attention to our intuition and act on what we hear or feel, we reduce stress and create more balance in our lives. The key here is not just getting the message, but listening to it and acting on it. According to Nancy Rosanoff, author of *Intuition Workout*, one study asked divorced couples when they first realized the relationship wasn't going to work out, and an astounding 80% replied, "Before the wedding." Although something told them that the marriage was foolhardy, each couple stood together at the altar, either because they wished too strongly that their intuition was wrong, or they didn't identify the message as a kind of knowing they could trust.

So how can we develop the intuitive side of our being? The best way is just to sit still and listen. Turn within and pay attention. Too often we run away from ourselves, filling up our lives with constant, stress-filled activity. We don't take time to be still. Often creative geniuses report that their "real world" discoveries are nothing other than self-discoveries from a deep silence within. When someone asked William Blake where he got his ideas, he replied that he stuck his finger through the floor of heaven and pulled them down. Michelangelo spurned the congratulations that were proffered him after having turned a block of stone into a sculpture of a man by saying the man was in there all the time and just required a little help in getting out. Franz Kafka wrote: "There is no need to leave the house. Stay at your desk and listen. Don't even listen, just wait. Don't even wait, be perfectly still and alone. The world will unmask itself to you, it can't do otherwise. It will rise before you in raptures." There is a profound benefit to hitting the pause button on your life every so often to create mini-respites, enabling you to connect with your inner silence and power.

Intuition can be nurtured in a variety of ways—through prayer and meditation, contemplation, walks in nature, or time spent alone gazing out a window or thinking. The more you act on your intuitive hunches, the stronger and more readily available they become. As you become more sensitive to your oneness with Jesus, Spirit, God, and life, you will become more intuitive.

Part of receiving those inner messages clearly comes when you learn to give up the analyzing, reasoning, doubting, and limiting part of your mind. Practice makes perfect. And intuition is infallible when you anchor yourself in the consciousness of the Divine. In *The Tao of Pooh*, Benjamin Hoff shares: "The masters of life know the Way. They listen to the voice within them, the voice of wisdom and simplicity, the voice that reasons beyond cleverness and knows beyond knowledge.

That voice is not just the power and property of a few, but has been given to everyone." And it was Helen Keller who gave us the following sagacious advice: "The most beautiful things in the world cannot be seen or even touched. They must be felt with the heart."

How can you simplify your life so that what's really important—what's really essential to live fully and celebrate life—can be uncovered and nurtured?

Also, where can you find ways to lift up other people in your life and bring them some simple joy? It could start with something as uncomplicated as being a good listener or giving someone a much-needed hug. As Joyce Meyer suggests to us in one of her motivating talks, "Encourage everyone you meet with a smile or compliment. Make them feel better when you leave their presence and they will always be glad to see you coming."

After reading through all of these tips and the pages of this book, think about what changes you are willing and eager to make in your new enriched lifestyle. It's time for commitment and when putting your goals down on paper, rather than simply keeping them in your mind and thoughts, they become more powerful. Use the space in the next chapter to write them down or photocopy the page and write them on the copy to post where you can see them often.

Let us be grateful to people who make us happy; they are
the charming gardeners who make our souls blossom.
~Marcel Proust

One can live magnificently in the world,
if one knows how to work and how to love.
~Leo Tolstoy

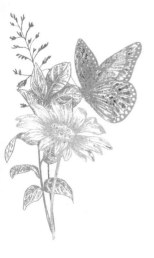

Chapter 15

Being Committed to Creating an Extraordinary Life

*The relationship between commitment and doubt is by
no means an antagonistic one. Commitment is healthiest
when it's not without doubt but in spite of doubt.*

~Rollo May

*Whatever you can do or dream, begin it!
Boldness has genius, power, and magic to it.*

~Johann Wolfgang von Goethe

Commitment Time

Here are some changes and choices I _____
(insert your name) will make this week, this month, and this year to
support my goal of creating a renewed life of vitality and purpose. I now
choose vibrant health and commit to living a balanced life.

This week:

1. _____

2. _____

3. _____

4. _____

5. _____

6. _____

7. _____

This month:

1. _____

2. _____

3. _____

4. _____

5. _____

6. _____

7. _____

This year:

1. _____

2. _____

3. _____

4. _____

5. _____

6. _____

7. _____

Personal Notes and More Good Intentions:

Signature: _____ Date: _____

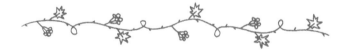

*The quality of a person's life is in direct proportion
to their commitment to excellence, regardless
of their chosen field of endeavor.*

~VINCE LOMBARDI

*The best way for us to keep fit and healthy is for us to
watch what we eat and think. Our choices of thoughts
and food are the major parts of either poor health or good
health. Life has given us unlimited choices and it's up to
us to educate ourselves on what really works for us.*

~LOUISE L. HAY

Part 6

When You Are Green Inside, You Are Clean Inside

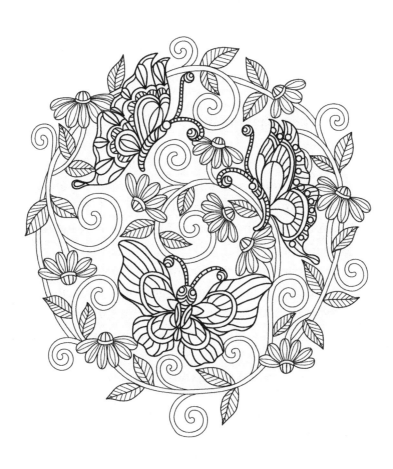

Chapter 16

Blending Your Way
to Radiant Well-Being

*I look younger. My skin is more supple now, and I
have fewer wrinkles than I did before eating raw.*

~Carol Alt

Live your life while you have it. Life is a splendid gift.

~Florence Nightingale

*A*s I've mentioned previously, *it's the little changes in your diet and
lifestyle that make the big difference in the long run.* Adding easy-
to-make, nutritious smoothies is a great place to start. In previous chapters, I recommended some of my favorite fruits and vegetables. If you
haven't read those parts, you might want to peruse them now before you
start experimenting with these recipes. And I do mean *experimenting*.
You can't go wrong when you make smoothies; they are among the
easiest and most delicious ways to ensure nutrient-bountiful meals.

Before I start with the smoothie suggestions and recipes, I wanted
to share with you an excerpt from the foreword for my book *Choose to
Thrive* by David Craddock. He describes a situation that occurred when
I was making a green smoothie recipe for one of my cooking classes I
taught in my home. It might make you laugh, too.

In every encounter Susan has with others, she always tries to build
someone up and find a way to tickle their funny bone. People tell
me often how good they always feel in Susan's presence. She's a

practical joker, yes indeed, and loves to laugh a lot. Susan taught me early on when I first worked with her about the power of relaxation to rejuvenate and restore the soul, the therapeutic effects and relationship-enhancing qualities of sharing fun and enjoyment together, and how we need to smile and laugh more, and she is the perfect example. Very little in life makes Susan upset and feel totally stressed out. Her attitude is always about seeing the best in everyone and everything and finding reasons to laugh as much as possible. No wonder her nickname is "Sunny." Let me give you one of many countless examples of Susan's jovial, comical, and light-hearted attitude . . . no matter the circumstances.

She was giving a cooking class to about 20 people in her home. This was the first class since she totally refurbished her kitchen and large adjoining family room with new cabinets, wood floors, shiplap on the walls, new paint everywhere, wood beam ceilings, new area rugs, etc.—everything was new and beautiful and she was so excited for her guests to see how she decorated it all.

It happened to be St. Patrick's Day and during this lunch-time class, everything was laid out on the massive marble island in the center of her kitchen and the guests were either seated around the island or standing behind. All of the foods we had made during the previous hour were displayed on the island for us to eat shortly. But first, she wanted to finish her cooking and nutrition demonstrations by making a healthy and delicious green smoothie. So into the blender went fresh almond milk (that was just made earlier), frozen blueberries and raspberries, a frozen banana, one cucumber, a tablespoon of flaxseeds and chia seeds, some baby leaf spinach, celery, a dash of cinnamon, and ice cubes. She blended it all in the 72-ounce jar, which was filled to the brim with scrumptious, creamy, totally blended green smoothie. She took off the lid and was about to give us all a sample when she realized that she forgot to put in some kale. Susan then asked one of the guests seated at the end island stool to get the kale from the refrigerator and finish making the smoothie while she went to use the bathroom and quickly changed her clothes before eating.

So while Susan was at the far end of her home in her bedroom suite, this guest put some kale into the blender and you've probably already guessed what was about to happen next. She forgot to put the lid on the blender after the kale went in and she pressed the start button, which was already set on high speed, before anyone had a chance to tell her to put the lid back on top first. With the force of an angry volcano, this green 72-ounce smoothie shot up to the high ceiling above, drenching all the shiplap in "green goodness" and also covering the entire island with all of the food, the floors, the area rugs, the walls, and most of the people watching, too. Everyone was in shock and didn't even know what to say so most of the guests were totally silently and, at the same time, very nervous because Susan's kitchen and family room was just refurbished and now everything was green.

Susan danced out of her bedroom and down the hall singing a song and was eager to sit down with everyone and start eating all of the foods that were just created the previous hour. Then she saw what happened and everyone was staring at her and Susan, to the surprise and delight of everyone, started laughing so hard that everyone else started laughing. It definitely relieved the tension in the room. But Susan couldn't stop laughing for about three minutes; in fact, she was laughing so hard that she was tearing up. Then she said joyfully, "It's my fault, I forgot to tell you to put the lid on, and how beautiful is this! Today is St. Patrick's Day and now there's no need to decorate because everything is already green." Well, that made all of the guests laugh even more. Everyone joined in with the cleaning up and Susan turned on some great music and ordered some food to be delivered from a local vegan restaurant for everyone to eat together, since all of the dishes/meals on the island ready to sample and eat were covered in green smoothie.

That, in a nutshell, is Susan. She's filled with vitality, joy, happiness, optimism, and celebration for everyone she meets and for life itself. And that's what shines through in the pages of this book, *Choose to Thrive*.

On to the Smoothies

Here are some suggestions you might want to experiment with in your smoothie adventures. I encourage you to make at least one green smoothie every day, and drink at least two cups. I usually average between two and four cups of green smoothie daily. Sometimes they are midmorning or midafternoon snacks, and sometimes they are my main meal, especially when I am in a rush and don't have time to make much more than a delicious, nutritious smoothie.

For the smoothies that follow, I combine a liquid base with approximately 30 to 40% fruit and 60 to 70% leafy and other greens. Find the percentages that appeal to your taste buds the most and especially to your intuitive side that wishes for more greens. In the forthcoming recipes, I've added in a little more fruit than I usually choose to put in a smoothie. You can always add in extra leafy green. To increase the nutritional benefit, I sometimes also add other vegetables such as baby carrots, bell peppers, or sprouts. If you notice that your smoothie is too thick, just add more liquid; if it's not sweet enough, add a date or other suggested sweetener. If it's not green enough, you can add a few more leaves of romaine lettuce or other leafy green.

When possible, go for all raw (and organic) ingredients as another way to increase nutritional value. The smoothie I make the most often combines pears, romaine or spinach (or both), alkaline water (or half water and half raw almond milk), a dash of cinnamon, and a coin of ginger root. That's it! It takes about three to four minutes to make, including the cleanup of the blender.

I encourage you to become a smoothie culinary expert. Get your family involved, too. Kids love to make smoothies and always enjoy the taste. It's such a great way to consume more greens without really tasting them. Enjoy!

Recommended Smoothie Ingredients

To prepare you to start making the smoothie recipes in the following chapter, here are the ingredients I recommend:

- **LEAFY GREENS AND OTHER VEGETABLES**: romaine lettuce, red leaf, Bibb, spinach, collards, Swiss chard, kale, arugula, watercress, beet greens, butter leaf lettuce, sunflower seed sprouts, or other wild or cultivated greens. Also try tomatoes, cucumbers, bell peppers, celery, fennel, squash, jicama, dandelion, burdock root, chicory, artichoke hearts, broccoli, beets, cabbage, cauliflower, corn, daikon, radish, sweet potato, yams, green onions, and sweet onions or shallots. (romaine lettuce leaves, especially the smallest ones, have the most neutral taste of all the leafy greens, and they add lots of nutritional value. I go through a head of romaine each day just for myself, and use this leafy green most often in my green smoothies.)

- **FRUITS**: Pears, apples, mangoes, blueberries, raspberries, cherimoya, grapes, apricots, strawberries, blackberries, cherries, cranberries, bananas, pineapple, papaya, lemons, limes, peaches, plums, nectarines, mulberries, kiwi, tangerines, persimmons, pomegranates, grapefruit, blood oranges, oranges, tangelos, and fresh figs.

- **THICKENERS**: Ice; young coconut meat; fresh figs; bananas (fresh or frozen); soaked dried fruits such as apples, dates, apricots, pineapple, cherries, papaya, and pears; nuts such as almonds, Brazil, macadamia, pecans, pine nuts, pistachio, walnuts, and cashews; raw nut butters such as almond, cashew, hazelnut, hemp, and macadamia; seeds (soaked and rinsed when appropriate) such as flax, chia, hemp, pumpkin, sesame, and sunflower; oils such as almond, coconut, flaxseed, grape seed, hemp seed, and olive (only for those you would like to put on some weight); miso—mellow yellow or mellow white work best with fruit combinations.

- **LIQUIDS AND JUICES**: Of course, this will vary depending on whether you're making fruit smoothies that include leafy greens such as romaine (they'll still taste like fruit smoothies), or you are making vegetable smoothies. Choose from any of the following liquids: purified water; freshly brewed teas such as peppermint, lavender, detox, lemon grass, green, white, black, or literally hundreds of other individual or combination herbal teas; freshly made juices from your juicer; store-bought nutritious juices such as cranberry, cherry, raspberry, blueberry, kombucha, pomegranate, coconut water, mango nectar, and papaya nectar; nut milks such as almond, cashew, macadamia, hemp, and walnut; and rice milk, oat milk, and banana milk.

❧ **SWEETENERS**: Pitted dates, bananas, date sugar, raw agave nectar, maple syrup, stevia (liquid or powder), raw honey, rice syrup, Sucanat, Sweet Leaf Organic Stevia, and other natural sweeteners. I encourage you to refrain from adding any sweetener until the end of the blending since fruit is usually sweet enough alone. Also, start to reeducate your taste buds and get used to the natural sweetness of fruit without adding extra sweeteners. (Only occasionally, I use pitted dates from time to time to sweeten or a banana.)

❧ **FLAVOR ENHANCERS AND SUPPLEMENTS**: Black cherry concentrate, tart cherry concentrate, coconut, pure vanilla extract, raw dark chocolate powder, and raw carob powder; edible essential oils such as cinnamon, ginger, fennel, and mint; flower essences such as orange blossoms, rose petals, and lavender; mixed dried fruits; cinnamon and nutmeg powders; wheatgrass juice; herbs such as oregano, rosemary, sage, and basil; ginger root; sea vegetables such as powdered dulse, kelp, and nori; lemon or lime zest; and even chili peppers, cayenne pepper, and hot sauce.

> *There is one thing on which most athletes and experts*
> *seem to agree. If you want to be an elite athlete, good*
> *nutrition at a young age is an important place to start.*
> ~CHUCK NORRIS

> *I'm healthy as can be—not an ache or a pain.*
> *A lot of my prayer is thanking the Lord that I am*
> *healthy. I pray for long life and good health.*
> ~JOEL OSTEEN

Chapter 17

Making Salubrious
Green Smoothies & More
That Everyone Will Love

I rely on a lot of green drinks to get my vegetables.

~TIM TEBOW

*When you feel great, you emanate a certain energy
that translates as beautiful. I don't care if you have the
standard beauty or not; it's that X-factor that comes
through, and the basis of that is good health.*

~CHRISTIE BRINKLEY

The following delicious smoothies are quick and easy to make. They are the ultimate "fast food." All you have to do is put the ingredients into a high-quality blender (adjusting the amount of liquid, if necessary) and *blend!* After just a week or two of making these fabulous smoothies (and the ones you dream up), you'll become a consummate smoothie aficionado and chef. Ladies and gentlemen . . . "Start your blenders!"

PEAR-KALE-MINT SMOOTHIE

3 pears

4 to 5 kale leaves

½ bunch fresh mint

¼ cup water

Place the ingredients in a blender with some of the water. Blend, adding additional water if necessary.

MANGO-PARSLEY SMOOTHIE

2 large mangoes

1 bunch parsley

¼ cup water

Place the ingredients in a blender with some of the water. Blend, adding additional water if necessary.

PEACH-SPINACH SMOOTHIE

5 to 6 peaches

2 cups spinach leaves

¼ cup water

Place the ingredients in a blender with some of the water. Blend, adding additional water if necessary.

BOSC PEAR-RASPBERRY-KALE SMOOTHIE

3 Bosc pears

½ cup raspberries

4 to 5 kale leaves

¼ cup water

Place the ingredients in a blender with some of the water. Blend, adding additional water if necessary.

BLUEBERRY-CELERY-ROMAINE SMOOTHIE

1 cup blueberries	4 romaine lettuce leaves
1 stalk celery	¼ cup water

Place the ingredients in a blender with some of the water. Blend, adding additional water if necessary.

APPLE-BERRY-SUNFLOWER SEED GREEN SPROUTS-KALE SMOOTHIE

1 apple	2 kale leaves
¾ cup raspberries (or other berries)	¼ cup water
1 cup sunflower seed green sprouts	

Place the ingredients in a blender with some of the water. Blend, adding additional water if necessary.

MANGO GREEN SMOOTHIE

1 cup fresh or frozen mango	4 to 5 romaine lettuce leaves
1 tablespoon raw macadamia butter	1 cup fresh apple juice
2 tablespoons flaxseed meal	(or other liquid)

Place the ingredients in a blender with some of the juice or liquid. Blend, adding additional juice or liquid if necessary.

BERRY GREEN SMOOTHIE

½ cup frozen raspberries	2 teaspoons flaxseed meal
½ cup frozen blackberries	5 to 6 romaine lettuce leaves
½ cup frozen strawberries	or 2 cups baby leaf spinach
1 teaspoon organic lemon zest (rind)	1 cup peppermint tea

Place the ingredients in a blender with some of the tea. Blend, adding additional tea if necessary.

SUNSHINE SMOOTHIE

1 cup frozen pineapple

1 frozen banana

½ cup fresh grapefruit juice

1½ cups torn kale leaves

3 to 4 romaine leaves

1/3 cup sunflower seed sprouts (optional)

1½ cups fresh orange or tangerine juice

Place the ingredients in a blender with some of the juice. Blend, adding additional juice if necessary.

PRUNE GREEN SMOOTHIE

5 soaked prunes

6 walnuts

2 teaspoon flaxseed meal

½ banana

4 romaine lettuce leaves or 1 cup of baby leaf spinach

¾ cup prune soaking water

Place the ingredients in a blender with some of the soaking water. Blend, adding additional soaking water if necessary.

V-8 GREEN SMOOTHIE

½ cup fresh celery juice

3 baby carrots

1 tomato

1 green onion

½ unwaxed cucumber

2 cups baby leaf spinach

3 romaine leaves

1 small red, yellow, or orange bell pepper

1 garlic clove (optional)

Dash of Celtic Sea Salt

1 cup fresh carrot juice

Place the ingredients in a blender with some of the juice. Blend, adding additional juice if necessary.

PERSIMMON GREEN SMOOTHIE

1 ripe persimmon

¼ cup pumpkin seeds

2 soaked figs

½ banana

2 medjool dates, pitted

2 cups romaine lettuce leaves or Swiss chard (or other leafy green)

Dash of cinnamon powder

½ cup fig soaking water

Place the ingredients in a blender with some of the soaking water. Blend, adding additional soaking water if necessary.

APPLE GREEN SMOOTHIE

1 cup apple slices

1 tablespoon raw almond butter

1 tablespoon raw hemp seed

1 cup leafy greens

¼ teaspoon nutmeg powder

¾ cup water or tea

Place the ingredients in a blender with some of the water or tea. Blend, adding additional water or tea if necessary.

PAPAYA GREEN SMOOTHIE

1 cup fresh or frozen papaya

½ cup pineapple juice or papaya nectar

1 teaspoon mellow white miso (or sweet miso of choice)

1½ cups leafy greens

Dash cinnamon

¼ cup raw aloe juice

Place the ingredients in a blender with some of the juice. Blend, adding additional juice if necessary.

FRUITY GREEN SMOOTHIE

2 tomatoes

2 peaches, sliced and frozen

2 plums, sliced and frozen

½ cucumber, diced

4 to 5 romaine lettuce leaves
or other leafy greens

½ cup water or other liquid

Place the ingredients in a blender with some of the water/liquid.
Blend, adding additional water/liquid if necessary.

CITRUS GREEN SMOOTHIE

1 grapefruit, peeled and quartered

2 oranges (or tangerines),
peeled and quartered

2 tomatoes

5 to 6 romaine lettuce leaves
or other leafy greens

¼ teaspoon cinnamon powder
(optional)

½ cup water or other liquid

Place the ingredients in a blender with some of the water/liquid.
Blend, adding additional water/liquid if necessary.

APRICOT-PLUM GREEN SMOOTHIE

3 large apricots

3 plums

6 romaine lettuce leaves
or other leafy greens

1 teaspoon lemon zest

Dash cinnamon powder

1 cup water or other liquid

Place ingredients in a blender with some of the water/liquid.
Blend, adding additional water/liquid if necessary.

KIWI-APRICOT GREEN SMOOTHIE

3 kiwis

5 apricots

¾ cup cucumber, sliced

2 sprigs parsley

2 kale leaves, spines removed

3 romaine leaves

1 tablespoon flaxseed meal

1 teaspoon lemon zest

1 to 2 medjool dates, pitted

2 cups water or tea

Place the ingredients in a blender with some of the water or tea. Blend, adding additional water or tea if necessary.

ORANGE-BERRY GREEN SMOOTHIE

2 cups raspberries

1 cup strawberries

1 orange, peeled

6 romaine lettuce leaves

1 teaspoon lemon zest

½ cup water or other liquid

Place the ingredients in a blender with some of the water/liquid. Blend, adding additional water/liquid if necessary. (With less water/liquid, it's a great chilled soup.)

BLUEBERRY GREEN SMOOTHIE

2 cups blueberries

3 large kale leaves, spine removed

2 to 3 medjool dates, pitted

¼ teaspoon vanilla extract

1¾ cups water or other liquid

Place the ingredients in a blender with some of the water/liquid. Blend, adding additional water/liquid if necessary.

RASPBERRY GREEN SMOOTHIE

2 cups raspberries

5 romaine lettuce leaves

2 medjool dates, pitted

1 teaspoon lemon zest

1 cup water

Place the ingredients in a blender with some of the water. Blend, adding additional water if necessary.

DETOX GREEN SMOOTHIE

1 grapefruit, peeled

1 orange, peeled

1 lemon, peeled

2 cloves garlic

1 tablespoon hemp or flaxseed oil

1 teaspoon minced fresh ginger

¼ teaspoon cinnamon

¼ teaspoon (or more) cayenne pepper

Place the ingredients in a blender, and blend. (The juices from the citrus make it the right consistency for me; if you want it thinner, simply add in some water, detox tea, or other liquid).

PEACH-BERRY GREEN SMOOTHIE

1 cup frozen berries (any type)

1 cup peaches, fresh or frozen

1 banana, fresh or frozen

2 cups leafy greens

15 to 20 almonds

2 teaspoons flaxseed meal

¼ teaspoon cinnamon

Pinch grated fresh ginger root

1½ to 1 cup water, tea, or other liquid such as coconut water

Place the ingredients in a blender. Blend, adding additional liquid if necessary.

TROPICAL GREEN SMOOTHIE

1 cup pineapple chunks

2 mangoes, peeled

1 papaya, seeded and peeled

2 cups leafy greens, chopped

½ cup sunflower green sprouts (optional)

1/3 cup pineapple juice or papaya/mango nectar

Place the ingredients in a blender with some of the juice or nectar. Blend, adding additional juice or nectar if necessary.

CARROT-APPLE GREEN SMOOTHIE

1/3 cup fresh celery (or fennel) juice

2 apples

1 tablespoon raw cashew
or almond butter

¼ teaspoon vanilla extract

¼ teaspoon minced ginger root

1 teaspoon lemon zest

3 sprigs parsley

¼ cup cucumber

¼ cup basil

1½ cups leafy greens

1 cup fresh carrot juice

Place the ingredients in a blender with some of the juice. Blend, adding additional juice if necessary.

COCONUT GREEN SMOOTHIE

1 cup young coconut meat

3 medjool dates, pitted

8 to 10 romaine lettuce leaves
(or butter leaf)

1 sprig parsley

1/8 teaspoon vanilla extract

¼ teaspoon lemon zest

3 cups coconut water

Place the ingredients in a blender with some of the coconut water. Blend, adding additional coconut water if necessary.

PURPLE-GREEN SMOOTHIE

1½ cups blackberries

3 medjool dates, pitted

1 banana

6 to 7 romaine, bibb,
or butter leaf leaves

¼ teaspoon lemon zest

1½ cups coconut water

Place the ingredients in a blender with some of the coconut water. Blend, adding additional coconut water if necessary.

PINK & GREEN LEMONADE

1 cup fresh orange juice

½ cup lemon juice

½ cup strawberries

5 to 7 hearts of romaine lettuce leaves

¼ teaspoon lemon zest

2 cups water

Place the ingredients in a blender with some of the water. Blend, adding additional water if necessary. (For Limeade, replace the lemon juice and zest with lime.)

FRESH PEACHY GREEN LEMONADE

3 lemons, peeled and seeded

½ cup raw agave (or raw honey), to taste

2 peaches, pitted

5 to 7 hearts of romaine lettuce leaves

Dash of cinnamon (optional)

4¼ cups purified water

Place the ingredients in a blender with some of the water. Blend, adding additional water if necessary.

SUNNY'S LUSCIOUS SWEET GREEN SMOOTHIE

1 pear, cored

12 frozen or fresh strawberries

2 bananas

1 lemon, peeled and seeded

1 medjool date, pitted

1/3 cup juice of blueberry, pomegranate, raspberry, açai, passion fruit, or combination

1 teaspoon cherry concentrate (optional)

6 to 8 hearts of romaine lettuce leaves

¼ cup apple juice or peppermint tea

Place the ingredients in a blender with some of the juice or tea. Blend, adding additional juice or tea if necessary.

FRESH FIG-KIWI GREEN SMOOTHIE

4 large fresh figs

2 large kiwi

3 cups romaine or hearts of
romaine lettuce leaves

¼ teaspoon cinnamon

1 teaspoon lemon zest

4 cups water or chilled chamomile
or peppermint tea

Place the ingredients in a blender with some of the water or tea.
Blend, adding additional water or tea if necessary.

NUT-NOG GREEN SMOOTHIE

¼ cup medjool dates, pitted

3 bananas

10 to 12 hearts of romaine
lettuce leaves

½ teaspoon nutmeg

1 teaspoon cinnamon

1 teaspoon vanilla extract

1/8 teaspoon turmeric

4 cups almond milk
(see Almond Milk to follow)

Place the ingredients in a blender with some of the almond milk.
Blend, adding additional almond milk if necessary.

ALMOND NUT MILK

1 cup raw almonds, germinated
(soak for 6 to 8 hours,
then rinse/drain)

3 to 4 cups purified water

1 tablespoon raw agave or other
sweetener (such as pitted dates)
(I don't use a sweetener)

Blend the almonds and water until the almonds are pulverized. If
using a sweetener, add it during the last few seconds of blending.
Strain through a cheesecloth, nut milk bag, or fine-mesh strainer
and discard the solids. Refrigerate.

SUSAN'S FAVORITE ALMOND-PECAN COMBO NUT MILK

½ cup raw almonds

½ cup raw pecans (a delicious antioxidant-rich nut)

3½ to 4 cups water

Soak nuts overnight in water. Drain and put into the blender with fresh water and blend for 60 seconds on high. Strain through a nut milk bag. (You can find these at health food stores or online.)

Variations: I often add a few drops of pure vanilla extract and/or a dash of cinnamon powder.

60-SECOND ALMOND MILK

2 tablespoons raw almond butter

1 teaspoon sweetener

A couple drops of vanilla extract (optional)

1 cup purified water (more or less for desired thickness)

Place the ingredients in a blender with some of the water. Blend, adding additional water if necessary.

VANILLA CHIA SEED PUDDING

This is so easy to make; it supports vitality and weight loss; and everyone loves it!

Serves: 2 to 4 (Depending on if it's a snack, dessert, or meal replacement)

4 tablespoons whole chia seeds

1½ cups almond milk (you can also use coconut, cashew, hemp, soy, oat, or rice milk)

2 tablespoons maple syrup (you can also use other liquid sweeteners

like agave or honey; I often don't use any sweetener at all)

¼ teaspoon pure vanilla extract (I often add in a few vanilla beans into the mixture, too)

7 to 12 whole almonds, chopped

Combine the ingredients, except the chopped almonds, thoroughly in a glass container and let sit in the refrigerator for at least 4 hours or overnight (best). When ready to eat, put the pudding in a transparent glass or other container and top with chopped almonds; I also often top with fruits (like berries), other nuts, or granola.

Hint: If you prefer a firmer consistency, add more chia seeds and less nut milk. Also, it takes about two minutes to make this pudding before bedtime, and it will be ready for your breakfast in the morning after chilling overnight in the refrigerator. Can't get much easier than this!

Variations: The sky's the limit with what you can add to the pudding recipe. I often cut open a vanilla bean and scrape out the seeds to mix in the pudding. (Did you know that vanilla is the second-most expensive spice after saffron?) Another favorite of mine is to add sliced bananas and blueberries with the vanilla seeds. Strawberries are wonderful in this pudding and so is a combination of banana slices, cut up figs, and strawberries. A sprig of mint always looks spectacular placed on the top of the pudding. I also like to put some fresh raspberries in the pudding. Experiment with the recipe and see what inspires your taste buds.

GOLDEN MILK

"Golden Milk" is a beautiful, tasty, and incredibly healthy drink especially suitable for drinking in the evening, and the benefits are outstanding (see page 254). This is a delicious nondairy way to get your daily turmeric and more!

Step 1: Turmeric Paste

¼ cup turmeric powder   ½ cup filtered water
½ teaspoon freshly ground pepper

Mix all the ingredients in a small cooking pot and stir well. Turn the heat to a medium and mix constantly until the mixture becomes a thick paste. It does not take a long time, so do not leave the stove. Let the mixture cool off, and then keep it in a small, covered jar in the refrigerator. I usually make it every week or two. It will last at least two weeks.

Step 2: Golden Milk

1 cup of almond milk (hemp milk or coconut milk are also a good option)

1 teaspoon of coconut oil

¼ (or more) teaspoon of turmeric paste (I use about 1 teaspoon or more)

Raw honey (optional; you can also use maple syrup, date sugar, stevia)*

I don't use any sweetener.

Mix all the ingredients in a cooking pot, except the honey. Turn the heat to medium. While you are heating the mixture, you must stir constantly and do not let it boil. Add honey according to your taste. I use my raw almond milk and don't heat it over 110°F to keep the enzymes intact.

Variations: Sometimes I'll sprinkle in some powder of cinnamon, cardamom, cloves, or sea salt in Step 2 and perhaps even some cayenne and/or ginger powder to give it more pizzazz and nutritional heftiness. On occasion, I blend a frozen banana to make it more like a Golden Milk smoothie. I might even add in an organic, raw sweet miso paste at the end to bolster the nutritional benefits even more. (I always have many different kinds of miso on hand in my refrigerator.) I drink it in a mug or glass although at times I put it in a bowl to enjoy as soup.

THE BENEFITS OF TURMERIC

The main ingredient in Golden Milk is turmeric. The turmeric contains curcumin, a polyphenol identified as the essential active ingredient, which reaches over 150 potential therapeutic activities, and includes antioxidant, anti-inflammatory, and anti-cancer properties. In combination with black pepper, the benefits of the curcumin increase considerably. By adding black pepper into dishes seasoned with turmeric, the bioavailability of curcumin is increased by about 1,000 times due to the piperine, the pungent property of black pepper. Yes, you read it right—by mixing the turmeric and the black pepper together, the body absorption of turmeric is increased to 2,000%!

Here are some of the additional advantages of turmeric:

* Anti-inflammatory, antioxidant, antiseptic, analgesic, and anti-carcinogenic activity

* Strengthens the immune system

* Helps maintain cholesterol levels

* Improves the digestive health

* Detoxifies the liver

* Beautifies skin

* Supports vision

* Regulates metabolism and controls weight

* Lowers high blood pressure

* Improves memory and brain function

* Remedies various skin conditions

* Protects against neurological disorders

* Reduces triglycerides

NATURAL HAND SANITIZER

Fritzie, my grandmother, would always insist that when I entered her home, I needed to wash my hands well in her kitchen before walking into any other room. To this day, I still do the same thing in my home and in other people's homes, too. Together, as a project, we also used to make natural hand sanitizers to give away as gifts. She was always decades ahead of anyone else when it came to healing the body and staying healthy—her healthy living practices. She was brilliant and full of joy.

Here is her wonderful and easy-to-prepare hand sanitizer recipe to use when you are not able to access soap and water. I spray it on my hands and also a variety of surfaces. If you want it thicker, use more aloe vera gel and funnel it into a squeeze bottle. For decades, I have purchased empty bottles at stores (clear or in different colors) to keep on hand for making these hand sanitizer gifts easily and quickly to give away and use myself. If I'm giving one as a gift, I might write on the bottle the three or more ingredients, or if it's, say, just lavender, I'll simply write: Susan's Natural Lavender Hand Sanitizer.

2/3 cup 60-90% rubbing alcohol (isopropyl alcohol)

1/3 cup aloe vera gel (you can find this in natural food stores or online)

3 to 8 drops essential oil (optional)*

In a bowl, mix these ingredients together (I use a whisk) and pour into your clean spray bottle. I usually use a funnel so I don't lose any of the mixture. If you are giving these away as gifts, tie a pretty ribbon around the bottle with a bow. Everyone to whom you give these natural hand sanitizer bottles will love them and ask you for the recipe.

As Fritzie always used to remind me, "Cleanliness is next to godliness."

* Here are some of my favorite essential oils to use: Tea Tree, Rosemary, Eucalyptus, Lavender, Grapefruit, Lemon, Basil, Chamomile, Ginger, Juniper Berry, Lime, Rose, Jasmine, and Olbas. Use them individually or mix two or three together such as Grapefruit, Lemon, and Lime. I purchase my essential oils at PennHerb.com—where I have been shopping for my natural products for decades.

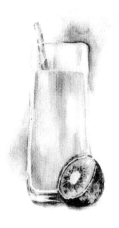
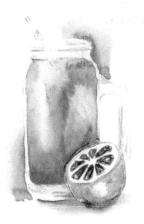
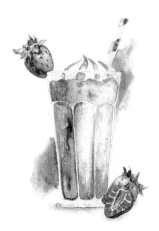

A lot of parents ask me how to get kids to eat more vegetables.
The first thing I say is that it starts from the top.

~Emeril Lagasse

We often forget that everything we see, animate or inanimate,
is a visual manifestation of the work of our invisible God.
We have become so accustomed to trees, mountains, sky,
air, water, flowers, animals, vegetables and people that
we no longer see them for what they are—God's work.

~Mother Angelica

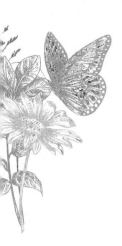

Chapter 18

Fast-Tracking Your Whole-Body Wellness with Super Greens

*In two decades I've lost a total of 789 pounds.
I should be hanging from a charm bracelet.*

~ERMA BOMBECK

*I feel an important part of beauty is not only what you
do on the outside but also what you put into the inside.
Good fresh food with many vegetables along with love
and caring for others. I spend way more time serving
others than I do on my beauty routine daily.*

~KIM ALEXIS

Throughout this book I have sprinkled in my love of greens to help in detoxifying the body and supporting high-level wellness, and now I will devote a chapter just to these gems of nature. Thirteen specific green foods can have a powerful effect on longevity and vitality. I will show you now how to attack aging—with your fork. If you want to live a long, vibrant life and up your odds of avoiding chronic disease, green and leafy vegetables should become an essential part of your daily diet. They provide a treasure trove of vitamins and minerals needed for a healthy immunity system. They also help ward off disease such as cancer. Leafy greens are excellent for the gallbladder, spleen, heart and blood, and are a good brain foods and natural laxative. Most greens can be cooked or eaten raw in salads or fresh juices. Most days I include greens in my smoothies (as I just covered in the previous chapter) and always in their raw form.

To clean your greens, separate the leaves and soak them in a sink of cold water and the juice of one lemon for a few minutes and swirl around, then drain the water. Pat or spin dry. Tear the leaves into small pieces, trim the ends of the stems and chop when necessary. All leafy greens contain chlorophyll, iron, magnesium, calcium, manganese, vitamin C, potassium, vitamin A, and a bonus of the essential fatty acids, with no cholesterol. The vegetables with the darkest, most intense colors tend to contain the highest level of nutrients. All lettuce is said to calm the nerves.

Here is a brief discussion of some of my favorite leafy greens:

■ ARUGULA

Also known as rocket, and from the mustard family, arugula is one of my favorite lettuce greens. It has a peppery and tart taste and mixes well with other greens. It adds pizzazz to any raw salad or sandwich, is high in vitamins A and C, niacin, iron, and phosphorus, and is good for normalizing body acid with its high alkalinity.

■ BEET GREENS

Best used in juices, beet greens are very high in nutrients, especially potassium, iron, and calcium. These greens also can be used in cooking. They are known for their benefit in blood disorders, liver function, and the flow of bile.

■ CHICORY

This is a bitter green with curly leaves; the young leaves are best in salads. Chicory is high in vitamins A and C, calcium, and iron and aids in liver function and blood disorders. Try radicchio, often called red-leaf chicory, which is great in salads and adds a stunning, beautiful color.

■ COLLARDS

This brilliant green vegetable is a member of the cabbage family. Use only the leaves. They tend to be tough, so you may want to steam them for a few minutes. Collards can be used in salads as a substitute for cabbage and are also great for juicing. Because of its high nutrient content, no leafy green is more valuable in the body for disorders of the colon, respiratory system, lymphatic system, and skeletal system.

■ DANDELION

Young dandelion leaves have a tangy taste. They are good for gall-bladder disorders, rheumatism, gout, and eczema and skin disorders. Dandelion is also an excellent liver rejuvenator. They cook the same as any leafy green. They are rich in calcium, potassium, and vitamins A and C. These are also excellent to add to juices.

■ ESCAROLE AND ENDIVE

From the chicory family, the leaves of escarole and endive are very dark green, with a slightly bitter taste. These make a good salad (with a citrus-flavored dressing) and also can be steamed. Both are rich in vitamin A, B vitamins, and minerals such as calcium, potassium, and iron. They're good for most infections, liver function, and internal cleansing.

■ KALE

Kale is the king of calcium. Use only the leaves of this plant unless juicing. It tastes like cabbage. I often add the juice of kale to carrot and other fresh vegetable juices. It's very high in usable calcium and is excellent for prevention and care of osteoporosis. FYI: a cup of kale surpasses the calcium content found in a glass of dairy milk and, because it contains an unusually high ratio of calcium to phosphorus, the calcium in kale is absorbed far more successfully.

■ MUSTARD AND TURNIP

These greens have a zippy taste with flavors varying from mild to hot. Both mustard and turnip greens are good sautéed with a little garlic or steamed, and also can be used in juices. They are high in calcium and vitamin C and are good for infections, colon disorders, colds, flu, and elimination of kidney stones due to excess uric acid.

■ PARSLEY

All types of this green herb are rich in vitamins A, B complex, and C, and minerals such as potassium and manganese. Parsley is very crisp and tangy. It is rich in chlorophyll, which provides a green "odor-eating" quality that helps restore fresh breath after a meal with such foods as garlic and onion. Add curly or flat-leaf parsley to fresh juice or chop and add to salads. It's good for digestive disorders and also an excellent diuretic.

■ ROMAINE

Romaine is a wonderful, crunchy green that is one of the highest in nutrients of all types of lettuce, including rich amounts of vitamins C and K. romaine is not recommended for cooking. Most days I put romaine leaves into my green smoothies. They are almost tasteless, contribute lots of fiber, and are excellent in smoothies for people who don't want any green taste. In the smoothies for children, these leaves are perfect.

■ SORREL

This green has a pleasantly sour and slightly lemon flavor. Sorrel is easily perishable and best bought fresh or grown in your garden. Try sorrel in salads or as a seasoning in soups and casseroles. Sorrel is a powerful antioxidant with the same healing properties as kale.

■ SPINACH

Its tender, bright green leaves are most beneficial when eaten raw. Because of the oxalic acid content in spinach, some of the calcium becomes unavailable to the body. Nevertheless, spinach contains many valuable nutrients and is high in chlorophyll, potassium, and iron.

■ SWISS CHARD

From the beet family, this green has a mild taste and is good with walnuts or pine nuts added to a salad. Swiss chard has the highest sodium content of all greens. Chlorophyll- and calcium-rich, Swiss chard is a natural cleanser and helps strengthen bones. Look for Swiss chard in red, green, and rainbow colors.

5 GOOD REASONS TO EAT YOUR GREENS

The more greens you eat, the better. Studies prove that people eating diets high in fruit and vegetables will always have a lower risk of heart disease, cancer, and diabetes, plus better memory and eyesight. Those are five excellent reasons to get the 5 to 9 servings you need.

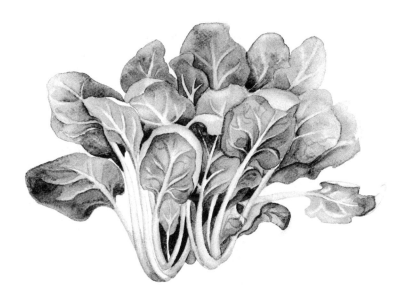

He who distinguishes the true savor of his food can never be a glutton; he who does not cannot be otherwise.

~Henry David Thoreau

Eat to live, don't live to eat; many dishes, many diseases.

~Benjamin Franklin

Afterword

Thoughts to Inspire
as You Transform Your Life!

*I believe that a simple and unassuming manner of life is
best for everyone, best both for the body and the mind.*

~ALBERT EINSTEIN

*You have to accept whatever comes and the only
important thing is that you meet it with courage
and with the best that you have to give.*

~ELEANOR ROOSEVELT

At birth, each of us is given the divine gift of laziness—the extremely important survival instinct to conserve energy. This conservation-of-energy instinct helped us survive in the millennia before the wheel, running water, electricity, and the disposable diaper. Of necessity, we mastered the art of weighing the risks and efforts required to attempt something against the potential benefits of succeeding at it. In simple terms, we learned not to "waste our valuable time or energy" unless we thought it was "worth it."

Changing your diet, making new shopping and kitchen habits, being more physically active, upgrading your lifestyle to emphasize high-level wellness, and learning how to be the "new you" in environments that are not always supportive can require considerable effort. Don't let your instinctive drive to conserve energy interfere with your desire to be all you can be.

I'm concluding this book with more of my favorite quotes to uplift you and help you focus on the deeper meanings of life and the joys of dedicating your life to them. George Bernard Shaw, never a man to mince words, put it this way:

This is the true joy in life, the being used for a purpose
recognized by yourself as a mighty one . . . being a
force of Nature instead of a feverish selfish little clod
of ailments and grievances complaining that the
world will not devote itself to making you happy.

The quotes to follow have inspired me over the years, and I hope that they will inspire you, too. There are even some lined, blank NOTES pages in the back of the book where you can add in your favorite quotes or other thoughts and ideas on how you are going to reinvigorate, renew, and rejuvenate your healthy living program and life.

Best wishes as you begin your personal journey to the mountaintop of high-level wellness!

Jesus himself stood among them,
and said to them, "Peace to you!"
~LUKE 24:36

What lies behind us and what lies before us are
small matters compared to what lies within us.
~RALPH WALDO EMERSON

We need to find God, and He cannot be found in noise
and restlessness. God is the friend of silence.
~MOTHER TERESA

Wake at dawn with a winged heart and give
thanks for another day of loving.
~KAHLIL GIBRAN

Of course I love everyone I meet. How could I fail to?
Within everyone is the spark of God. I am not concerned
with racial or ethnic background or the color of one's
skin; all people look to me like shining lights!

~PEACE PILGRIM

For as he thinks in his heart, so is he:

~PROVERBS 23:7

It is a great relief when for a few moments in the
day we can retire to our chamber and be completely
true to ourselves. It leavens the rest of our hours.

~HENRY DAVID THOREAU

Be joyful in hope, patient in affliction, faithful in prayer.

~ROMANS 12:1

I submit that scientists have not yet explored the hidden
possibilities of the innumerable seeds, leaves, and fruits
for giving the fullest possible nutrition to mankind.

~MAHATMA GANDHI

Hope is the thing with feathers
That perches in the soul
And sings the tune with words
And never stops at all.

~EMILY DICKINSON

Faith is the confidence that what we hope for will actually
happen; it gives us assurance about things we cannot see.

~HEBREWS 11:1

Write it on your heart that every day is the best day of the year. He is rich who owns the day, and no one owns the day who allows it to be invaded with fret and anxiety.

~RALPH WALDO EMERSON

No matter what will be said and done, preserve your calm immovably; and to every obstacle, oppose patience, perseverance, and soothing language.

~THOMAS JEFFERSON

So, as those who have been chosen of God, holy and beloved, a heart of compassion, kindness, humility, gentleness, and patience.

~COLOSSIANS 3:12

If we did all the things we are capable of doing, we would literally astound ourselves.

~THOMAS EDISON

If your daily life seems poor, do not blame it; blame yourself that you are not poet enough to call forth its riches; for the Creator, there is no poverty.

~RAINER MARIA RILKE

God sees every single thing we do, and if we can keep the right attitude and the right serving heart, God will supply everything we need. Our job is to keep the faith.

~LAURIE CROUCH

For I have plans for you. Plans to prosper you and not to harm you, plans to give you hope and a future.

~JEREMIAH 29:11

If you look at what you have in life, you'll always have more.
If you look at what you don't have, you'll never have enough.

~Oprah Winfrey

Kites rise highest against the wind—not with it.

~Winston Churchill

You weren't created to be a mud pot. God made
you to be a golden vessel, so live accordingly.

~2 Timothy 2:20

Some people seem to think that my life dedicated to
simplicity and service is austere and joyless, but they do
not know the freedom of simplicity. I am thankful to
God every moment of my life for the great riches that
have been showered upon me. My life is full and good
but never overcrowded. If life is overcrowded then
you are doing more than is required for you to do.

~Peace Pilgrim

Nothing will benefit health and increase the chances for
survival of life on Earth as the evolution to a vegetarian diet.

~Albert Einstein

The trustworthy person will get a rich reward, but a
person who wants quick riches will get into trouble.

~Proverbs 28:20

Invite Jesus to make an indelible impact on your heart and in
your life. Just your willingness to open up to His Light and
Love is a simple step that will reward you monumentally.

~Susan Smith Jones

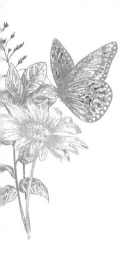

Gratitudes

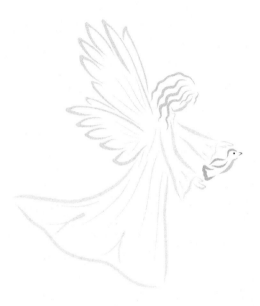

Devote yourself to prayer, being watchful and thankful.

~Colossians 4:2

*Cultivate the habit of being grateful for every good thing
that comes to you, and to give thanks continuously.
And because all things have contributed to your advancement,
you should include all things in your gratitude.*

~Ralph Waldo Emerson

As I strive to live my dream with as much heart, grace, and gratitude as possible, there are many people who have enriched my life and helped me to create this positive, informative, and beautifully designed book.

No book is ever written by the author alone. I am indebted to so many whose names may not be mentioned—most especially the people who have come to my talks and workshops worldwide over the years and have helped me to refine the *modus operandi* and information contained within. They encouraged me to be courageous and share some of my private and personal stories about my life's challenges and adventures, which I always discuss in my talks. Many of my clients have also given me permission to include narratives about their life lessons to help bring more joy and inspiration to the pages of this book.

To my shepherd, Christ Jesus, and my guardian angels—who nurture my spiritual side, enrich my life, and guide me along this magnificent journey with their gentle touch, wise counsel, and loving presence. Thank you for being the wind beneath my wings and showing me that all challenges can be overcome and that dreams can become reality with enough love, faith, and patience. Highlighting Psalm 23, I know without any doubt that my absolute trust in Christ gives me grace and mercy all the days of my life, restores my soul, and leads me beside still waters. With a heart filled with gratitude, I dwell in the house of the Lord forever.

With a heart full of gratitude, I also thank David Craddock, who inspires me with his positive attitude about life, never-ending generosity, strong integrity, and delightful sense of humor; and for motivating and encouraging me to write this book—as he wrote about in the foreword. An eternal optimist, David knows me exceedingly well, and it was his insight into me and what he believes the world needs to learn more about in order to achieve high-level wellness that stimulated him to suggest my writing this book.

> *"The optimist sees opportunity in every danger;*
> *the pessimist sees danger in every opportunity.*
> *A pessimist sees the difficulty in every opportunity;*
> *an optimist sees the opportunity in every difficulty."*
>
> ~ SIR WINSTON CHURCHILL

To Ginny Swabek, who is a dear, most-cherished friend and has been like a sister to me for decades. Thank you for being an earth angel in my life, for always being my best support, for encouraging me to stay focused on this book and my life's goals, for reading many of the pages of this book and other work I do and proffering feedback and editing suggestions, and for bringing so much joy and comfort into my life.

To my sisters, Jamie and June, I give my deepest gratitude for being two more earth angels in my life—for always giving me their unconditional love and support, and believing in me when I didn't believe in myself.

To all my earth angels who were pleased to contribute their endorsements, I thank you immensely. All of these wonderful people and friends have inspired me in countless ways. They include Myran Thomas; Brian Boxer Wachler, MD; Peter W. Brown, MD; Nancy S. Schort, DDS; Rev. Brittian Bowman; Ric Bratton; Olin Idol, ND, CNC; Angie Dunkling Averill, DMD; Gordon Averill, DMD; Nick Lawrence; Karla Calumet, PhD; and Finley W. Brown, Jr.

To the most wonderful couple I've ever had the pleasure of working with—Carol and Gary Rosenberg (TheBookCouple.com). Not only are they two of the most supportive, kind, and easy people with whom to work but, to boot, they are also experts at their profession. This angel husband and wife team undertook the task of editing this book, designing the delightful interior, creating the dazzling cover, helped me package the book so it could get to people worldwide, and so much more. In fact, they've helped me with all my books for my publishing company, Books To Uplift (BooksToUplift.com), cofounded with David Craddock. They are simply the best at their artistic craft, and I treasure my friendship with them both.

To you, dear reader, because you make a difference in the world. I pray that this book will renew your hope, inspire your soul, lift your spirit, make you think, and strengthen your resolve to live the life you've always wanted to live. You can be healthy, happy, and peaceful, and you can help to bring about a more peaceful, balanced world. You are important to the well-being of planet Earth.

Acknowledging the good that you already have in your life is the foundation for all abundance.

~ ECKHART TOLLE

Let gratitude be the pillow upon which you kneel to say your nightly prayer. And let faith be the bridge you build to overcome evil and welcome good.

~MAYA ANGELOU

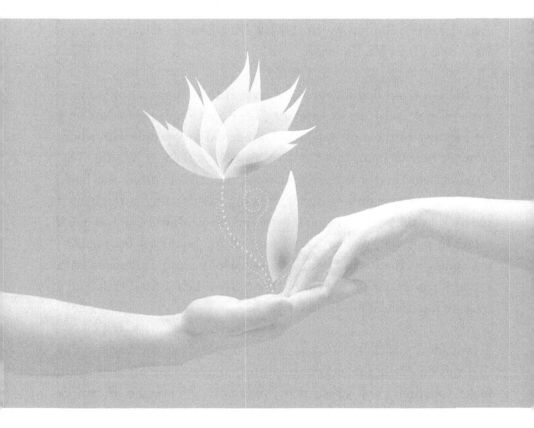

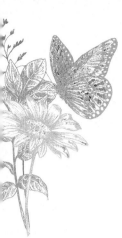

About
Susan Smith Jones, PhD

A cheerful heart is good medicine,
but a broken spirit saps a person's strength.

~PROVERBS 17:22

Why don't you start believing that no matter what you have or
haven't done, that your best days are still out in front of you.

~JOEL OSTEEN

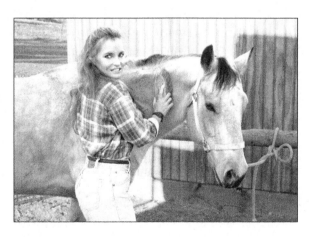

For a woman with three of America's and the UK's most ordinary names, Susan Smith Jones, PhD, has certainly made extraordinary contributions in the fields of holistic health, longevity, optimum nutrition, high-level fitness, and balanced, peaceful living. For starters, she taught students, staff, and faculty at UCLA how to be healthy and fit for 30 years!

Susan is the founder and president of Health Unlimited, a Los Angeles–based consulting firm dedicated to optimal wellness and holistic health education. As a renowned motivational speaker, Susan travels internationally as a frequent radio/TV talk show guest and motivational speaker (seminars, workshops, lectures, and keynote address); she's also the author of more than 2,500 magazine articles and over 33 books, including—*Invest in Yourself with Exercise; Be the Change, Kitchen Gardening, A Hug in a Mug, Choose to Thrive, and UPLFTED: 12 Minutes to More Joy, Faith, Peace, Kindness & Vitality.*

Susan is in a unique position to testify on the efficacy of her basic message that health is the result of choice. When her back was fractured in an automobile accident, her physician told her that she would never be able to carry "anything heavier than a small purse." Susan chose not to accept this verdict; within six months, there was no longer any pain or evidence of the fracture. Soon, she fully regained her health and active lifestyle.

Susan attributes her healing to her natural-foods diet, a daily well-rounded fitness program, a strong God- and faith-centered life, along with the power of determination, balanced living, and a deep commitment to expressing her highest potential. Since that time, she has been constantly active in spreading the message that anyone can choose radiant health and rejuvenation. Her inspiring message and innovative techniques for achieving total health in body, mind and spirit have won her a grateful and enthusiastic following and have put her in constant demand internationally as a health and fitness consultant and educator.

A gifted teacher, Susan brings together modern research and ageless wisdom in all of her work. When she's not traveling the world, she resides in both West Los Angeles and England.

If you enjoyed this book, please visit: **SusanSmithJones.com, ChristianLifestyleMatters.com** and **BooksToUplift.com** for more details on Susan and her work. Her books and websites are like having a "holistic health app" for anything related to holistic health and living a faith- and God-centered life.

If you'd like to receive Susan's free monthly *Healthy Living Newsletters* filled with uplifting, empowering, and high-powered information, go to **SusanSmithJones.com** and sign up on the page *Subscribe & Win!* It takes only 10 seconds and you will also receive several gifts from Susan.

Imagination is more important than knowledge.
For knowledge is limited to all we now know
and understand, while imagination embraces
the entire world, and all there ever will
be to know and understand.

~Albert Einstein

As you keep your mind and heart focused in
the right direction, approaching each day
with faith and gratitude, I believe you will be
empowered to live life to the fullest and enjoy
the abundant life He has promised you!

~Victoria Osteen

NOTES

Lead me in your truth, and teach me.

~Psalm 25:5

Create in me a clean heart, O God,
and put a new and right spirit with me.

~Psalm 51:10

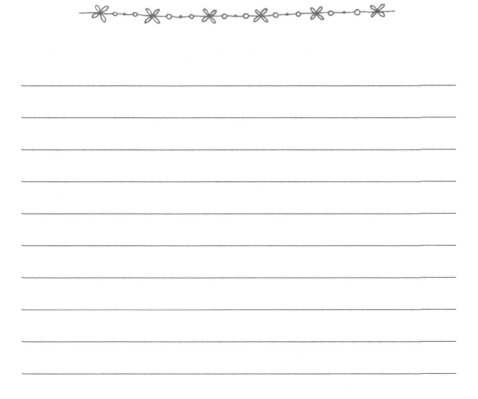

You will decide on a matter, and it will be established
for you, and light will shine on your ways.

~JOB 22:28

So let us not grow weary in doing what is right, for
we will reap at harvesttime, if we do not give up.

~GALATIANS 6:9